NEW DEVELOPMENTS IN MEDICAL RESEARCH

BURSITIS OF MAJOR JOINTS

NEW DEVELOPMENTS IN MEDICAL RESEARCH

Additional books in this series can be found on Nova's website under the Series tab.

Additional e-books in this series can be found on Nova's website under the e-book tab.

NEW DEVELOPMENTS IN MEDICAL RESEARCH

BURSITIS OF MAJOR JOINTS

ALESSANDRO APRATO
EDITOR

New York

Library of Congress Cataloging-in-Publication Data

ISBN: 978-1-63482-295-4
Library of Congress Control Number: 2015932990

Published by Nova Science Publishers, Inc. † New York

Contents

Preface

Bursitis knowledge continues to evolve. This book presents new technology and techniques related to this pathology and it reflects these exciting changes and new information. We divided it into five chapters according to the anatomical region. Each chapter has been further divided into seven paragraphs (introduction, anatomy, physiopathology, clinical evaluation, imaging, conservative treatment and surgical treatment) although some chapters present additional specific paragraphs. The scheme of chapter was designed to ensure that the most current detailed information is presented. For example, diagnosis is paramount in the care of those patients; in each chapter the authors describes the surgeon's roles to achieve a proper diagnosis. Physiopathology paragraphs deal with basic science aspects that are important to clinicians while surgical treatment paragraphs represent scientific advances in which surgeons are leading the charge. Finally the imaging paragraphs reflect the wider changes in the last two decades for the definition of the diagnosis and to choose the correct treatment.

The primary goal of this book is to be the most thorough, useful, readable, and understandable textbook describing major joint bursitis. It is designed to be equally useful to students, trainees, and experts in the field.

Alessandro Aprato

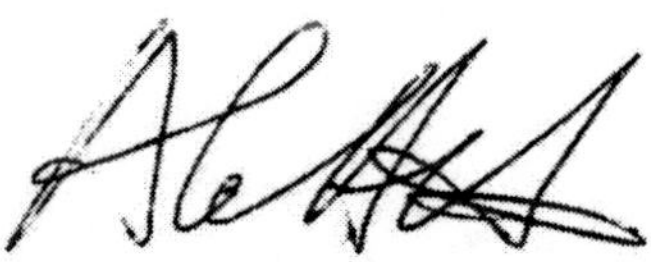

In: Bursitis of Major Joints
Editor: Alessandro Aprato

ISBN: 978-1-63482-295-4

Chapter I

Bursitis Around the Shoulder

Lorenzo Mattei[1]*, MD, Chiara Arrigoni[2], MD, Antonio Pastrone[1], MD, and Filippo Castoldi[1], MD, Prof

[1]University of Torino, Department of Orthopaedics and Traumatology, AO Città della Salute e della Scienza, Presidio CTO, Torino, Italy

[2]University of Torino, Department of Orthopaedics and Traumatology, Ospedale San Luigi di Orbasano, Torino, Italy

Abstract

Shoulder bursitis is one of the most common causes of shoulder pain, mostly caused by overuse of the joint or repetitive trauma on the shoulder. Its clinical importance is often overlooked, the diagnosis is confused with other diseases. In literature, there is no consensus on bursistis treatment, then its management is often based on surgeon's experience. The bursae of the scapulothoracic articulation are often the source of problems in the joint kinematics. Their inflammation are frequently misdiagnosed and not properly treated.

In this chapter we focus on the etiopathogenesis and anatomy of the many bursae of the glenohumeral and scapulorthoracic articulations.

We examine the entire diagnostic process, underlining the importance of an accurate diagnosis. We conclude by describing some

* Corresponding author. Via Zuretti 29, 10100, Torino, Italy. Email: lorenzo.mattei87@gmail.com

principles for therapy, and evaluate conservative treatments consisting of NSAID, physiotherapy, corticosteroids injections, and arthroscopic surgery.

Our goal is to highlight the important aspects of the disease, allowing the young doctor to face it more confidently, and to offer a detailed review to the more experienced reader.

Keywords: Shoulder, bursitis, scapula, anatomy

Introduction

Donald P Carpenter [1] said "The term bursitis, altough listed as diagnosis, still includes a number of clinical and pathological entities wich can and should be separated. The term bursitis often violates good medical practice by naming the symptom as a diagnosis. [...]. Bursitis is often a symptom... not a primary disease and hence not a proper diagnosis".

This text was published in 1958. By this time the MRI did not exist, orthopaedic knowledge was limited, and Neer's and Hawkins's tests were to be described only 20 years later.

In this chapter we will focus our attention on the anatomical, biological, functional and instrumental approach, as well as the conservative and surgical treatment.

Anatomy

The bursae are anatomical structures formed by a mesenchymal membrane similar to synovia, surrounding a viscous liquid. They are strictly connected to muscles, tendons and joints and they allow a smooth sliding of these structures between them.

Different kinds of bursae are contained in the shoulder, with a huge variability in composition and function. In particular subscapularis and bicipital bursa, contained in the shoulder joint, have a huge impact on the range of motion of the shoulder.

Other important bursae are the subacromial bursa (contained between the upper surface of the joint capsule and the lower surface of the acromion), the subcoracoid bursa (between the lower face of the coracoid and the joint capsule), and the coracobrachial bursa (between the conjoint tendon and the capsule joint) (Figures 1-2).

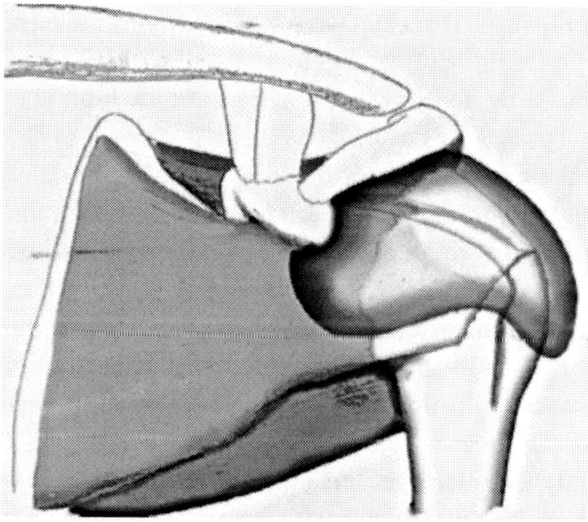

Figure 1. Schematic representation of subacromial bursa.

Teres major, latissimus dorsi (anterior and posterior), pectoralis major, infraspinatus (between the muscles and the posterior part of the scapular neck), and the subcutaneous acromial bursae are described as well [2].

The most important bursae are, however, the subscapularis and the bicipital ones, as they are strictly related to the capsule.

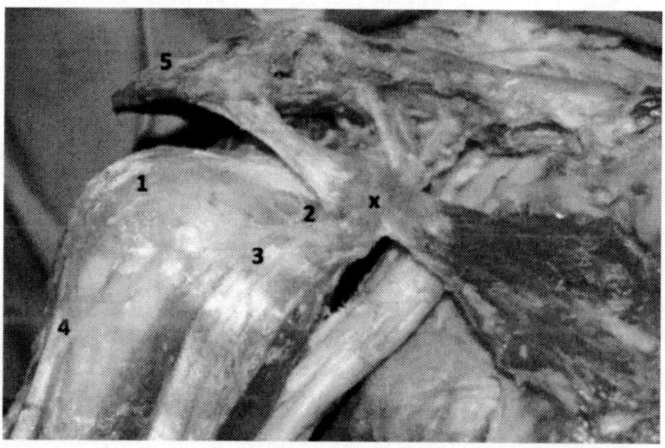

Figure 2. The anatomy of the bursae. 1 subacromial bursa, 2 subcoracoid bursa, 3 coracobrachial bursa, 4 bicipital bursa, 5 above acromion. X coracoid process.

The joint capsule communicates anteriorly with the subscapularis bursa, and inserts posteriorly and inferiorly on the edge of the glenoid labrum. In this region the joint can also communicate with the infraspinatus bursa.

Usually, the synovial tissue wraps the intra-articular part of the biceps brachialis tendon (long head) producing a tubular sheet that allows the sliding of the tendon upwards and downwards during abduction and adduction of the arm [3].

Clinically, the most important bursa is the subacromial one. It divides the two muscular layers that cover the lateral surface of the joint and allows their sliding, protecting the rotator cuff (deep plane) from the contact with the acromial bone, the coracoacromial ligament (who fills the gap between the coracoid process and the acromion) and the scapular coracoid process.

This bursa is a wide anatomical structure that extends itself to the lower portion of the coracoid process. In this site it allows the sliding between the conjoint tendon and the subscapular muscle.

In the healthy shoulder the bursa doesn't communicate with the inner part of the joint, however, it may occur with a tear in the supraspinatus tendon.

This bursa changes its anatomical position during the movement of the upper limb. It is normally placed just below the deltoid muscle and the coracoacromial ligament. When the upper limb is abducted the bursa moves under the coracoacromial ligament and is pressed between the lower surface of the acromion and the humeral head causing pain, especially if there is inflammation. The coracoacromial ligament usually hides the local tenderness, making diagnosis more difficult.

When the upper limb is placed forward, the pain disappears, as the bursa is no longer compressed; in this case there may be local tenderness on the lateral side, inferiorly to the acromion, because the bursa is now accessible to palpation [3].

It is mandatory to also consider the bursa located on the scapular-thoracic joint.

It differs from the other shoulder joints because it's composed from some muscle layers and by a bursa that allows the movements of the structures [4].

Wlliams et al. described three layers: the superficial (trapezius and latissimus dorsi muscles), the intermediate (rhomboid major and minor and elevator scapulae muscles) and the deep one (subscapularis and serratus anterior muscles) [5].

Kuhn et al. [6] reported the locations of six bursae (2 major, 4 minor) in the scapulothoracic joint. The scapulothoracic (infraserratus) and subscapularis (supraserratus) bursa, located in the deep layer, are considered primary physiologic bursae [5, 7, 8].

The subscapularis bursa is located between the subscapularis and serratus anterior muscle, and has an average area of 5,3 x 5,3 cm [5], while the infraserratus bursa is located under the serratus anterior and overlays the posterolateral chest wall and has an average area of 9,0 x 7,4 cm [5]. The other minor bursaes are often the result of abnormal scapulothoracic movement [7].

These are typically found along the inferior angle of the spine, at the superomedial border of the scapula, either above or below the serratus anterior, or deep to the trapezius muscle at the medial base of the scapular spine [9].

The bursa of the superomedial border and inferior angle frequently causes pain [10, 11].

An intermediate bursa, approximately 4,3 x 2,7 cm wide, named trapezoid bursa, is located between the superomedial scapular angle and the trapezius muscles [12].

Physiopathology of Bursitis

The term bursitis often describes a number of clinical and pathological entities: the primary bursitis, the cystic degeneration, the calcareous deposits, and the so-called "chronic sprains".

Actually, the term "bursitis" is used to identify a primary inflammation of a bursa. On the other hand, it is considered as a symptom if associated with another disease [1]. In those cases subacromial bursa inflammation may arise from autoimmune inflammatory conditions (rheumatoid arthritis), crystal deposits (Gout or Pseudo gout), calcific loose bodies (rheumatoid arthritis) and infection [13].

As in all inflammation processes, primitive bursitis is a pathological response of the body, and is caused by leukocytes and plasma proteins productions. The main causes of the acute form are the changes in blood flow, due to vasodilatation, and the increased vascular permeability to plasma proteins and leukocytes.

In case of bursitis, the cells tend to accumulate with their products in the cavities of the bursa, leading to exudate production (in case of high protein concentration) or transudate (in case of low protein concentration).

Bursitis may occur in an acute, subacute or chronic stage.

The chronic phase is due to the coexistance between tissue destruction and the attempt of the body to repair it.

It is typically characterized by an infiltration of mononuclear cells, tissue damage and stimulation of angiogenesis and fibrosis [14].

Subacute and chronic types of bursitis are recognized in both superficial and deep layers of the bursae. Thickening of the synovial wall and villous projections can occur. Only these types are defined bursitis [1].

Clinical Evaluation

Shoulder pain and dysfunction may result from various aetiologies and pathologies. A common cause is impingement (pinching), which causes 'catching' or pain without considerable joint stiffness.

In 1977 Neer and Welsh described the impingment as a pinching of the soft tissue between the acromial arch and humerus during movement [15]. More specifically, these soft tissue structures include the rotator cuff, the subacromial bursa and the biceps tendon.

A thorough clinical examination with an accurate patient's history can guide the physician to a precise diagnosis. Specific functional tests are to be executed only after a precise observation.

The examination begins by observing the patient's walk. The position of the upper limb, how the patient uses his arm to undress, if he uses walking aids such as crutches, are all factors that must be carefully considered.

For example, a patient with severe pain generally keeps the upper limb adduct, and often uses the other arm to support his weight. The movement of the whole upper body is often clumsy and not smooth, while the patient is undressing. Any deformity, muscolar or bony must be observed.

It is important to observe the profile of the deltoid on its three portions (anterior, middle and posterior), and to check the supraspinatus and infraspinatus. The atrophy of these last muscles can result in a prominence of the scapula and can be caused by an injury of the rotator cuff, by entrapment of the suprascapular nerve, or by myopathies. In particular, the atrophy of the supraspinatus results in an evident bone profile of the scapular spine.

Typically the subacromial bursa is not visible, but severe cases of rheumatoid arthritis, for example, can lead to its swelling. Often, in these cases, the bursitis is also visible due to the associated atrophy of the deltoid.

The patient should be questioned regarding the precise location, quality, and intensity of the pain. The patient's way of life should also be documented for appropriate goal setting.

Palpation

In order to diagnose bursitis and to exclude other diseases, it is important to palpate some important anatomical structure.

Subacromial bursa: the bursa should be palpated in all its extension, looking for thickening or masses, which can be felt with small movements, passive and active. The patient often complains of crackling sounds that may be related to bursal thickening. During passive extension of the shoulder, the bursa moves anteriorly to the acromion and becomes more easily palpable.

Bicipital groove: bordered by the greater tuberosity and the small tuberosity of the humerus, it is the seat of the LHB. In case of inflammation or subluxation, the palpation of the sheath that covers the LHB causes pain. Palpation becomes easier with the limb in an externally rotated position.

Acromionclavicolar joint: sometimes the pain caused by a bursitis can be confused with the one caused by arthritis of the ACJ, especially when there is a chronic inflammation, and when the patient is unable to locate precisely the pain. The ACJ is easy to feel. The joint movement can be easily appreciated, flexing and extending the shoulder a few times. The presence of pain may be related to arthritis or dislocation of the lateral end of the clavicle.

Range of Motion

The evaluation of the active and passive range of motion is a complex but mandatory step in order to understand the shoulder's pathology. Usually the examinator asks the patient to move the arm in three diferrent directions, comparing the range of motion with the other arm. The abduction of the shoulder is better observed from posterior view, as it is for the observation of the scapulothoracic rhythm, that is harmonic in an unaffected patient. The painful arc test, defined as pain during active abduction, usually starts near 90° and sometimes disappears at full abduction, and is useful to identify impingment in general terms [16]. Calis et al. [17], have described a specificity of 82% to target subacromial and internal impingment for this test, but low sensitivity of 32%.

The evaluation of the active and passive external and internal rotation is important to exclude other pathology such as the frozen shoulder.

When the internal rotation is analyzed with the Scratch Apley test, asking the patient to bring the hand to the back, it is important to keep in mind that the glenohumeral rotation contributes for only 2/3 of the range of motion, and the reached level is influenced by the elbow flexion. [18].

To assess scapular impingment, an accurate evaluation of the scapulothoracic rhythm as well as its protraction and retraction, is necessary. In a snapping scapula syndrome, the alternation of protraction and retraction determines a palpable squeak, sometimes audible, usually detectable at the superomedial angle of the scapula.

Specific Tests

When a person presents a history of shoulder impingment or subacromial bursitis, the clinician performs a series of physical tests that aims to estabilish the diagnosis.

Many tests have been described by several authors to identify impingment syndrome and subacromial bursitis. The current literature doesn't focus on subacromial bursitis as a single entity and is often associated with subacromial impingement; furthermore, most of the studies focus on tests for rotator cuff thears, overlooking the importance of impingment and bursitis.

From different studies and reviews analyzed, the results of many tests have been shown to differ with examiner experience [19, 20, 21, 22].

Calis et al. [17] have reported an high specificity (97%) for the combination of all tests used for the diagnosis of subacromial impingment, but very low sensitivity (only 5%): this last data means tests are rarely all together positive, because they all investigate different aspects of the same disease.

The test described by Hawkins and Neer, is widely used by clinician all around the world, but there are some others tests that could be useful in less clear situation:

Neer Sign

The tester elevates the sitting patient's arm, preventing scapular movement by pressing down on the clavicle and acromion with the other hand. The sign is positive if this manouver provokes pain. The sign have a good sensitivity (89%) but low specificity (32%) [17]. Others authors revealed that the sensitivity and specificity for the Neer test were respectively 72% and 60%

[19]. The test is furthermore confirmed when the patient is given an injection of 10 ml, 1% xylocaine beneath the anterior acromion before the monouver is repeated. A positive Neer's sign shows no more pain [23]. With this last procedure, the test shows a lower sensitivity (75%) and higher specificity (48%) [24] (Figure 3).

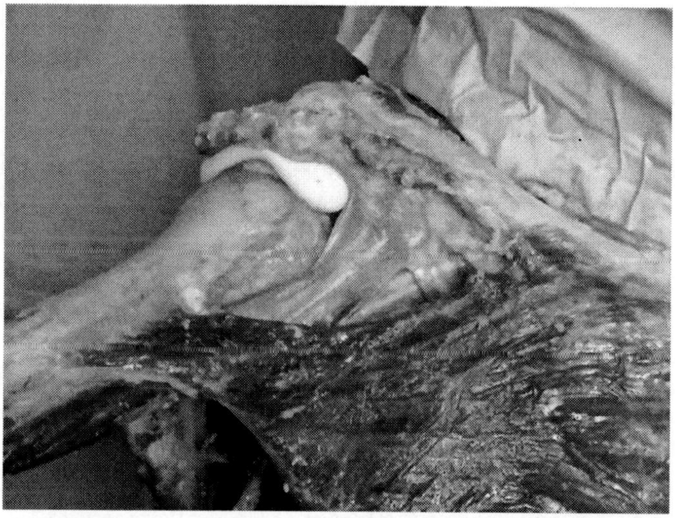

Figure 3. The subacromial bursa is represented here with a balloon (cadaveric model).

Hawkins Test

Both shoulder and elbow of the affected limb are placed at 90°. The tester then medially rotates the patient's shoulder. The test is positive when it provokes pain [25].

Fodor et al. reported that the Hawkins-Kennedy test is the most sensitive test for identification of subacromial impingement syndrome, whilst Neer's test is the most specific [26]. Other authors report that Hawkin's test has a higher diagnostic odd ratio than the Neer sign (5.18 vs 3.83) [19].

Yokum Test

This test was described for the first time by Naredo, who misinterpreted a photograph illustrating Hawkin's test. The patient places the hand of the affected arm on his controlateral shoulder and raises the elbow of the affected limb. The test is positive when the movement reproduces patient's pain [27]. According to Naredo et al., the combination of Hawkins' test, Neer's sign, and

Yocum's test seems to have a good sensitivity (0.43 [0.18, 0.71]) and excellent specificity (0.88 [0.64, 0.99]).

Gum Turn Test

The test is performed in the standing position with the involved arm in an abducted position of 90°, with anteposition and external rotation of the limb. The patient is then invited to reproduce a spiral movement on a drawing sheet for 20 turns. The test is considered positive when the patient is not able to achieve it due to strength decrease or to shoulder pain [28]. The test resulted hardly reliable as a detector of subacromial impingement or as a detector of small cuff tear. When the test is positive there is a high probability that a subacromial disease exists; on the other hand, a negative test shows a high probability that the patient has not a massive cuff tear.

Calis et al. [17] investigate the diagnostic values of clinical tests, in patients with a subacromial impingement syndrome. A high sensitivity in Hawkins test (92.1%), Neer test (88.7%) and horizontal adduction test (82.0%) was found. Tests with the highest specificity were the drop arm test (97.2%), Yergason test (86.1%) and painful arc test (80.5%). They conclude that diagnostic tests are insufficient for certain diagnosis.

It is not always simple to differentiate between symptoms of subacromial bursitis, or of the long head of the biceps (LHB) inflammation. To investigate the LHB, different tests and signs could be performed. The palm up test, described for the first time by Gilcreest [29] in 1936, is positive in case of frequent dislocation of LHB tendon. The patient should elevate the arm with the hand supinated, holding a weight in the hand. The tester palpates the LHB while the patient tries to resist the lowering of his arm. The test is positive when a definite snap is audible and/or palpable, and a sharp pain is provoked both in the shoulder and in the region of the bicipital groove. Speed's [30] and Yergason's [31] test are more specific in detecting an inflammation of the LHB. In the first one, the patient *flexes* his shoulder against *isotonic resistance* with the elbow extended and the forearm *supinated;* in the second the patient's elbow is *flexed* to 90° and the forearm *pronated.* The patient then actively *supinates* against resistance. Both the tests are positive in case of pain in the region of the bicipital groove.

To asses tendons or muscle rupture, lag signs [32, 33] and specific tests could be performed to describe accurately wich tendons are affected and to which extent [21].

Scapolothoracic Bursitis

Patients with scapulothoracic bursitis or snapping scapula usually complain of pain, scapular noise, and/or crackling sensations with the arm movement, especially with overhead activities [4, 34,]. Each one of these symptoms can vary [4, 35] in intensity. In addition to that, it is important to investigate a possible acute traumatic event causing their discomfort [36].

It is known that significant kyphoscoliosis reduces scapulothoracic congruence and may induce scapular snapping with or without painful bursitis [6, 37], that's why an evaluation of the posture and of the cervical-thoracic spine should be performed in all patients. In case, differential diagnosis should be excluded, investigating pain syndrome resulting from nerve compression [38] or enlarging tumors that push the scapula away from the posterior thorax [6].

Bilateral inspection of both shoulders, focused on asymmetry, audible snapping, winging, is then performed. It is important to bear in mind that overhead sport athletes will often have depression, protraction, and downward rotation of their dominant scapula, without any relation with their primary complaint [39].

Scapular winging is a common finding in patients with scapulothoracic bursitis and may be the result of a abnormal periscapular muscle kinematics such as weakness or tightness of the serratus anterior, trapezius, levator scapulae, and/or pectoralis minor muscles.

Palpation around the scapulothoracic articulation may reveal areas of localized tenderness, corresponding to infraserratus or supraserratus bursal inflammation. Sometimes, patients can reproduce movements that generate scapulo-thoracic crepitus. In these cases, it is often helpful to palpate the scapula during active motion to localize the site of inflammation [4]. Placing the arm in the ''chicken wing'' position (the humerus is internally rotated, and the dorsum of the hand is placed over the lumbosacral junction) may help tilting the scapula laterally, allowing deeper palpation beneath the medial scapular border [9]. By applying posterior-to-anterior pressure over the scapular body during range of motion, the tester can also value crepitation between the scapula and the posterior thorax and may reproduce the patient's symptoms [40].

Individual periscapular muscle strength testing should also be performed to identify any points of weakness that may result in scapular dyskinesia and subsequent bursitis or snapping. Trapezius muscle strength can be evaluated by simply having the patient shrug the shoulders while the clinician applies resistance. The strength of the elevator scapulae and rhomboid musculature is tested by having the patient place the hands on the ipsilateral iliac crests and retracting the scapula by moving the elbows posteriorly. Resistance of this motion can also be performed to assess corresponding muscle strength. The serratus anterior muscle is tested by having the patient perform a wall push-up while the examiner simultaneously visualizes and palpates the medial border of the scapula. Serratus anterior weakness would most likely result in medial scapular winging during this test. The latissimus dorsi muscle is tested by having the patient press posteriorly against resistance with the arms at the side while also palpating the inferomedial angle of the scapula [41].

Imaging

X-Ray

Plain radiographs are usually normal in impingment syndrome, especially in acute phase. However, true anteroposterior, tangential Y, and axillary views have to be obtained to investigate painful shoulder. They may demonstrate subacromial spurs, acromion abnormalities, calcifying tendinitis or other skeletal abnormalities that could contribute to understand the biomechanical mechanism of subacromial or scapulothoracic bursitis.

Blonna et al. [42], have described the “critical shoulder angle” (CSA) formed by the tangential line of the glenoid and the line from the inferior pole of the glena to the lateral extremity of the acromion. It was calculate that normal patients have a CSA of 33.8°. A higher CSA mostly correlates with a cuff tear arthropathy and angles inferior to 28° seem to correlate with the development of concentric arthritis. No statistical correlation was found with the CSA and the development of subacromial bursitis or calcification.

However, these lesions are not always visible on the X-ray, especially when lesions are of soft tissue or are not sufficiently calcified. Some authors suggest using fluoroscopy to dynamically identify bony lesions, especially for scapulothoracic bursitis, but we believe this technique is unnecessary for the diagnosis and presents an increased radiation exposure [43].

Computed Tomography

In literature there are no evidence about the effectiveness of CT scan in diagnosis of subacromial bursitis. We think it could be useful if there are some bony anomalies.

Different authors have tried to evaluate the clinical utility of computed tomography (CT) to explore scapulothoracic crepitus [44, 45]. They found an excellent reliability, but findings on CT scans do not seem to correlate with clinical findings, especially when there is no skeletal lesion such as osteochondroma or scapulothoracic incongruity. Routine CT scanning is therefore not suggested in patients with scapulothoracic bursitis/crepitus without documentation of a bony or cartilaginous lesion. A CT scan with or withouth 3D reconstruction could be requested to better evaluate or characterized the lesions for the purpose of surgical planning.

Park et al. [46] propose 3-dimensional CT scanning as a method to quantify scapular dyskinesis. This study only accounts for changes in the resting position of the scapula.

Magnetic Resonance Imaging (MRI)

Magnetic resonance imaging (MRI) is generally regarded as the gold standard for shoulder imaging. It is well tolerated by patients and reliable in evaluating most clinical situations. It is a static examination, often requiring arthrography to optimise diagnostic accuracy in patients with subtle internal lesions, and may demonstrate “incidental” findings, leading to potentially mistaken diagnosis and useless additional investigations [47].

Nevertheless it has demonstrated its diagnostic utility in the subacromial space in which it has replaced the use of ultrasonography and arthrograms [48]. In subacromial bursitis MRI imaging can reveal fluid accumulation in the bursa. In chronic cases caused by impingement, tendinosis and tears in the rotator cuff may be revealed (figure 4).

Some authors believe that it is an excellent non invasive tool for the identification of some soft tissue lesions associated or not with cuff tear rupture, such as subdeltoid bursitis [49].

The MRI provides detail of potential sites of subacromial impingement through the supraspinatus outlet. Ossification of the coracoacromial ligament (CAL) or presence of a subacromial spur can be best identified in the sagittal oblique plane; however, differentiation of a pathological spur and the normal

CAL can be difficult. MRI also may show subacromial/subdeltoid bursitis. This condition is often revealed by bursal thickness >3 mm, presence of fluid medial to the acromioclavicular joint, and presence of fluid in the anterior aspect of the bursa [50].

Several authors [51, 52, 53, 54, 55] highlight the importance of MRI in the detection and characterization of soft tissue masses or tumors, cystic lesions and in the prevention of misdiagnoses and unnecessary surgical intervention.

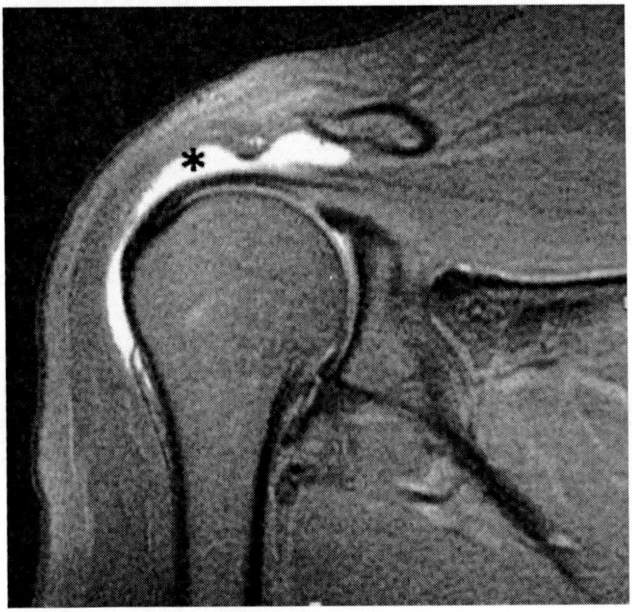

Figure 4. The subacromial bursa is clearly identifiable. It is noted that the inflammation extends to long head biceps tendon (MRI view).

Ultrasound

The subacromial-subdeltoid bursa usually appears, on the US, as a 2-mm-thick complex consisting of an inner layer of hypoechoic fluid between two layers of hyperechoic peribursal fat [56]. Fluids accumulate in the most declive portions of the bursae and, more commonly, along the lateral edge of the greater tuberosity, producing a typical "teardrop" appearance [56].

The term "bursitis" appears frequently in radiology reports of shoulder ultrasonography, implying a specific diagnostic entity, but the published literature contains no suitable definition of SAB on ultrasound [57]. By tacit consensus, the term "bursitis" appears to have become a description for bursae judged by the radiologist to contain excessive fluid or bursae with synovial or fibrotic thicken- ing. But an excessive amount of fluid in the subacromial bursa may result from its communication with the glenohumeral joint caused by tear in the rotator cuff, or from bursal impingement with an intact rotator cuff. Thickening of the subacromial bursae may result from chronic bursal impingement or may be physiological, reflecting the protective function of the bursae in upper limb athletics or in overhead worker. The lack of consensus in assessment of the subacromial bursa [58, 59] and the high incidence of "bursitis" in asymptomatic individuals [60, 61] suggest that attention is needed in interpreting SAB on ultrasonography [62].

Concerning the scapulothoracic bursitis, although ultrasound has been reported as a possible modality for the diagnosis of inflamed bursal tissue [63], it is most commonly used to guide needle placement for diagnostic and therapeutic injections [4, 64]. In general, the temporary resolution of pain after the injection confirms the diagnosis of bursitis and precisely localizes the pathological bursae.

Electromyograms

An electromyogram may become necessary in patients with unexplained scapular winging and/or periscapular muscle weakness. In particular, lateral scapular winging may be caused by atrophy or weakness of the serratus anterior muscle as a result of a long thoracic nerve injury. Medial scapular winging can be the result of trapezius muscle weakness due to a spinal accessory nerve dysfunction, which may be caused by an aberrant arthroscopic portal placed superior to the level of the scapular spine.

Therapy for Subacromial Bursitis

Nonoperative Treatment

The first approach to subacromial bursitis should be nonoperative. It initially consists of pharmacological treatment with non steroidal anti-inflammatory drugs, physical therapy and local injection into the inflamed bursa. The effectiveness of the instrumental therapy is still under debate.

The physical therapy for the treatment of the subacromial bursitis is strongly supported by the literature. Therapeutic exercises have been demonstated to improve the shoulder range of motion, the joint pain and the overall shoulder function during every day life. It has been shown to be more successful than no treatment or placebo, and it should be performed before any operative option in patients affected by subacromial bursitis [65].

Physical therapy basically consists of strenghtening the rotator cuff, the scapular stabilizator muscles, and of stretching the anterior and posterior shoulder girdle.

The anteposition of the shoulder is shown to be frequent in patients with subacromial bursitis after postural evaluation, and it is usually caused by a weak scapular stabilsation system.

Scapulo-toracic hypermobility provokes an early humerus-acromial arch impingement during arm elevation, for that reason the scapular stabilisation during every-day activities by strenghtening the scapular stabilizer muscles should be one of the most remarkable goal of the physical therapy.

Moreover, a stronger rotator cuff, obtained especially by focusing on exercises for the internal and external rotator muscles, prevents the migration of the humeral head towards the acromial arch. In consequence of this, the subacromial space during the range of motion is wider, avoiding early contact between the humeral bone and the subacromial arch [66].

Manual therapy, associated to physical therapy, improves the outcomes in patients treated for subacromial bursitis. A passive glenohumeral mobilisation combined to active exercises seems to be more effective that active exercises only, as it helps to recover the full range of motion by stretching the anterior and posterior capsule of the shoulder.

The treatment of the cervical and toracic spine and muscles by manual therapy was demonstrated to be an effective option, with significant improvement of the clinical outcomes. It proves that attention to the closer joints should be paid for a complete medical care.

Lastly, agopuncture seems to be useful in the management of short-term pain, but at now there are no significant long-term benefits.

Subacromial infiltrations with corticosteroid drugs are recognised to be an effective treatment for patients affected by subacromial bursitis. The injections can be really quick in reducing the shoulder pain, especially in patients who are unable to follow a physical therapy program. The subacromial space can be easily reached through a posterior or lateral way of access, depending on the experience of the surgeon. Some author advocate the use of ultrasound to guide the needle in to the inflammed bursa, as it is demonstrated to result in a significant improvement of the clnical outcomes, if compared to blind infiltrations [67].

Injections can also give some important information about the correct diagnosis when the clinical examination is limited by pain. If the pain disappears after the injection and the patient is able to actively abduct the arm, a subacromial bursitis is more likely the cause of the desease.

Corticosteroid infiltrations are potentially detrimental for the rotator cuff tendons, but the frequency and dose of injections necessary to provoke damage to the soft tissues are still unknown.

The effect of injections in patients affected by diabetes has been verified. After a single subministration of corticosteroid the growth of the blood glycemia is statistically higher but not clinically significant, if diabetes is well compensated [68, 69].

Surgical Treatment

Conservative, nonoperative management is often successful, but when it fails, surgical treatment should be taken into consideration.

There is no evidence that surgical treatment is superior to conservative approach, but usually most of the patients who undergo an operation have been previously unsuccessfully treated with injection or physical therapy, therefore a selection bias should be hypothesized. These findings strenghten the concept that surgery should be performed after an unseccessfull conservative treatment [70].

The aim of the subacromial decompression is the removal of the inflamed bursa, in order to give to the patient relief from pain [71].

An arthroscopic decompression should be preferred rather than open surgery because it is a less invasive procedure for the soft tissue [72].

Indeed, during the open technique the deltoid muscle is detached from its acromial insertion and it usually produces an early muscle weakening that can delay active mobilization of the shoulder after surgery [73].

The success rate of the arthroscopic subacromial decopression ranges between 77% and 90% and the major complication rate is less than 1 %. The most frequent complication is the brachial plexus neuropraxya, that can be easily prevented by avoiding traction of the arm during patient positioning [74].

For starting a simple arthroscopic decompression, standard anterior, posterior and lateral portal are needed for the insertion of the arthroscope.

After the identification of the anatomical structures, the bursa can be easily removed by motorized shaver or a monopolar radiofrequency cautery device. If the bursa is particularly inflamed, attention should be paid to the bleeding, as it can be difficult to interrupt, expecially for an inexperienced surgeon.

The effectiveness of acromioplasty for the treatment of subacromial bursitis is still controversial. This procedure is based on Neer's extrinsic impingement theory in which the inflamation of the bursa is caused by the contact between the inferior surface of the acromion and the subacromial tissues. The removal of the prominence from the anterior part of acromial bone results in a wider subacromial space, avoiding impingement of the tissues during the elevation of the arm [75].

The disadvantages of acromioplasty originate from the distruction of the coracoacromial arch, which represents a secondary stabiliser for the humeral head. This procedure can lead to anterosuperior instability and weakening of the deltoid origin. Furthermore the exposure of the bone of the inferior surface of the acromion can predispose to the development of adhesion on the rotator cuff tendon. The analysis of the shoulder anatomy through X-ray is mandatory before the decision making. Acromioplasty should be performed in case of acromion type III or II and after the evaulation of the width of the subacromial space.

Failure of subacromial decompression is generally due to incorrect indication or technical error and usually consists of lasting pain and shoulder instability [76].

Therapy for Scapulo-Toracic Bursitis

If mechanical incongruence, or lesions that can cause scapulo-toracic impingment, have been excluded, the first approach to snapping scapula syndrome is nonoperative.

The treatment consists of physical therapy focused on stabilising the scapula during the shoulder motion, and of modification of the altered posture with dedicated exercises. Simultaneous assumption of non steroidal anti inflammatory drugs has been demonstrated to improve the clinical outcomes [11].

Subscapular corticosteroidal and local anesthetics infiltration are valuable for the treatment and diagnosis of scapular bursitis. For an easier procedure, the bursa can be exposed by positioning the patient in the “chicken wing” position, with the arm internal rotated, adducted and extended. The needle must be inserted parallel to the scapular plane in lateral direction in order to prevent pneumothorax. Pain resolution after local anesthetic infiltration is a useful tool for the diagnosis confirmation of scapulo-toracic bursitis.

If conservative treatment doesn't solve the problem after some months of physical therapy, a surgical approach should be evaluated [77].

Operative treatments include open or arthroscopic bursectomy. The open option should be taken into consideration when a mechanical incongruence is thought to be the cause of the scapulotoracic impingement. The operation consist of an open partial scapulectomy of the superomedial angle. The resection is usually made with an oscillating saw after the exposure of the superomedial angle of the scapula. The bone edges left after the cut should be smoothed for warding off the risk of pain after surgery. If there is no evidence of mechanical scapulo-toracic impingement, open or arthroscopic bursectomy without scapulectomy are both viable options. During arthroscopic bursectomy the patient is positioned in the before mentioned "chicken wing" position for obtaining the best exposure of the scapulo-toracic space. Surgical accesses should be placed at least 2 cm to the medial border of the scapula for preventing damages of the dorsal scapular nerve. The removal of the inflamed bursa is generally performed with a motorized shaver device, but radiofrequency can be a valuable solution when bleeding is expected.

The rehabilitation program after arthroscopical bursectomy lasts for four week and consists of strenghtening of the scapular stabilizator muscle. The most frequent complications after surgery are the injury of the dorsal scapular nerve or artery, pneumothorax, injury of the long thoracic nerve, recurrence of the bursitis and haematoma.

The complication rate ranges from 5% to 29%, and for that reason attention should be paid to the patient selection.

References

[1] Carpenter DP. Bursitis; often and inexact diagnosis. *Calif Med.* 1958 Feb;88(2):151-4.

[2] Balboni C, Bastianini A, Brizzi E, Castorina S, Comparini L, Donato R et al. Anatomia Umana vol.1 Edi.ermes 3° edizione, ristampa aggiornata 2000, pp 57- 241.

[3] Hoppenfield S, DeBoer P. *Vie di accesso e anatomia chirurgica in Ortopedia.* Verduci Editore 3° edizione 2006, pp 21-38.

[4] Gaskill T, Millett PJ Snapping scapula syndrome: diagnosis and management. *JAAOS* 2013 vol. 21 no. 4 pp 214-224.

[5] Williams Jr GR, Shakil M, Klimkiewicz J, Iannotti PJ Anatomy of the scapulothoracici articulation. *Clinica Orthopaedics and related research* 1999 no. 359 pp 237-246.

[6] Kuhn JE, Plancher KD, Hawkins RJ. Symptomatic scapulothoracic crepitus and bursitis. *J Am Acad Orthop Surg.* 1998;6(5):267-273.

[7] Kuhne M, Boniquit N, Ghodadra N, Romeoand AA, Provencher MT The snapping scapula: diagnosis and treatment. *Arthroscopy* 2009 vol. 25 no.11 pp 1298-1311.

[8] Colas F, Nevoux J, Gagey O The subscapular and subcoracoid bursae: descriptive and functional anatomy. *Journal of Shoulder and Elbow Surgery* 2004 vol. 13 no. 4, pp 454-458.

[9] Millett PJ, Gaskill TR, Horan MP, Van der Meijden OA Technique and outcomes of arthroscopic scapulothoracic bursectomy and partial scapulectomy. *Arthroscopy* 2012 vol 28 no.12 pp 1776-1783.

[10] Ruland III LJ, Ruland CM, Matthews LS Scapulothoracic anatomy for arthroscopist. *Arthroscopy* 1995 vol 11, no 1, pp 52-56.

[11] Conduah AH, Baker Jr CL Clinical management of the scapulothoracic bursitis and the snapping scapula. *Sports Health* 2010 vol. 2 no.2 pp 147-155.

[12] Frank RM, Ramirez J, Chalmers PN, McCormick FM, Romeo AA Scapulothoracic anatomy and snapping scapula syndrome. *Anatomy Research International vol. 2013* Hindawi Publishing corporation pp 1-9.

[13] Salzman KL, Lillegard WA, Butcher. Upper extremity bursitis. *Am Fam Physician.* 1997 Nov 1;56(7):1797-806, 1811-2.

[14] Kumar V, Abbas AK, Fausto N et al. *Robbins e Cotran- Patholologic Basis of Disease* 7th edition. 2005, Elsevier Ed. pp. 49-85.

[15] Neer CS, Welsh RP. The shoulder in sports. *Orthopedic Clinics of North America* 1977;8(3):583–9.

[16] Cyriax JH. *Textbook of orthopaedic medicine: Diagnosis of soft tissue lesions.* 8th Edition. Vol. One, London: Balliere Tindall, 1982.

[17] Calis M, Akgun K, Birtane M, Karacan I, Calis H, Tuzun F. Diagnostic values of clinical diagnostic tests in subacromial impingement syndrome. *Annals of the Rheumatic Diseases* 2000;59(1):44–7.

[18] Mallon, WJ; Herring, CL; Salley, PI et al. Use of vertebral levels to measure presumed internal rotation at the shoulder: A radiographic analysis. *Journal of Shoulder and Elbow Surgery* 5: 299-306, 1996.

[19] Hegedus EJ, Goode AP, Cook CE, Michener L, Myer CA, Myer DM, Wright AA. Which physical examination tests provide clinicians with the most value when examining the shoulder? Update of a systematic review with meta-analysis of individual tests. *Br J Sports Med.* 2012 Nov;46(14):964-78. doi: 10.1136/bjsports-2012-091066. Epub 2012 Jul 7.

[20] *American Shoulder and Elbow Surgeons: Curriculum Guide for Treatment of Shoulder Injury.* http://www.ases-assn.org/?p=shoulder-curr.

[21] Hanchard NC, Lenza M, Handoll HH, Takwoingi Y. Physical tests for shoulder impingements and local lesions of bursa, tendon or labrum that may accompany impingement. *Cochrane Database Syst Rev.* 2013 Apr 30;4:CD007427. doi: 10.1002/14651858.CD007427.pub2.

[22] Dinnes J, Loveman E, McIntyre L, Waugh N. The effectiveness of diagnostic tests for the assessment of shoulder pain due to soft tissue disorders: a systematic review. *Health Technol Assess.* 2003;7(29):iii, 1-166.

[23] Neer CS 2nd. Impingement lesions. *Clinical Orthopaedics & Related Research 1983*;(173):70–7.

[24] MacDonald PB, Clark P, Sutherland K. An analysis of the diagnostic accuracy of the Hawkins and Neer subacromial impingement tests. *Journal of Shoulder and Elbow Surgery* 2000;9(4):299–301.

[25] Hawkins RJ, Kennedy JC. Impingement syndrome in athletes. *American Journal of Sports Medicine* 1980;8(3): 151–8.

[26] Fodor D, Poanta L, Felea I, Rednic S, Bolosiu H.Shoulder impingement syndrome: correlations between clinical tests and ultrasonographic findings. *Ortop Traumatol Rehabil.* 2009 Mar-Apr;11(2):120-6.

[27] Naredo E, Aguado P, De Miguel E, Uson J, Mayordomo L, Gijon-banos J, et al.Painful shoulder: comparison of physical examination and ultrasonographic findings. *Annals of the Rheumatic Diseases* 2002;61(2):132–6.

[28] Gumina S, Bertino A, Di Giorgio G, Postacchini F. A new test of resistance in the diagnosis of postero-superior rotator cuff tears. *Chir Organi Mov.* 2008 Feb;91(2):85-6. doi: 10.1007/s12306-007-0014-3. Epub 2008 Mar 3.

[29] Gilcreest EL. Dislocation and elongation of the long head of the biceps brachii: an analysis of six cases. *Annals of Surgery* 1936;104(1):118–38.

[30] Crenshaw AH, Kilgore WE. Surgical treatment of bicipital tenosynovitis. Journal of Bone & Joint Surgery - *American Volume* 1966;48(8):1496–502

[31] Yergason RM. Supination sign. *Journal of Bone and Joint Surgery - American Volume* 1931;13(1):160.

[32] Hertel, R; Ballmer, FT; Lambert, SM et al. Lag signs in the diagnosis of rotator cuff rupture. *Journal of Shoulder and Elbow Surgery* 5: 307-313, 1996.

[33] Castoldi F, Blonna D, Hertel R. External rotation lag sign revisited: accuracy for diagnosis of full thickness supraspinatus tear. *J Shoulder Elbow Surg.* 2009 Jul-Aug;18(4):529-34. doi: 10.1016/j.jse. 2008.11.007. Epub 2009 Feb 14.

[34] Burkhart SS, Morgan CD, Kibler WB. The disabled throwing shoulder: spectrum of pathology. Part III: the SICK scapula, scapular dyskinesis, the kinetic chan, and rehabilitation. *Arthroscopy.* 2003;19:641-661.

[35] Milch H. Snapping scapula. *Clin Orthop.* 1961;20:139-150.

[36] Carlson HL, Haig AJ, Stewart DC. Snapping scapula syndrome: three case reports and an analysis of the literature. *Arch Phys Med Rehabil.* 1997;78:506-511.

[37] Cobey MC. The rolling scapula. *Clin Orthop Relat Res.* 1968;60:193-194.

[38] Makin GJV, Brown WF, Ebers GC. C7 radiculopathy: importance of scapular winging in clinical diagnosis. *J Neurol Neurosurg Psychiatry.* 1986;49:640-644.

[39] Priest JD, Nagel DA. Tennis shoulder. *Am J Sports Med.* 1976;4(1): 28-42.

[40] Millett PJ, Pacheco I, Gobezie R, et al. Management of recalcitrant scapulothoracic bursitis: endoscopic capulothoracic bursectomy and scapuloplasty. *Tech Shoulder Elbow Surg.* 2006;7:200-205.

[41] Ryan J. Warth, Ulrich J. Spiegl and Peter J. Millett Scapulothoracic Bursitis and Snapping Scapula Syndrome: A Critical Review of Current Evidence. *Am J Sports Med,* March 24, 2014 DOI: 10.1177/ 0363546514526373.

[42] Giani A., Assom M., Caranzano F., Rossi R., Castoldi F., Blonna D. Studio dei fattori di rischio per le patologie degenerative di spalla. Poster session SICSeG 2014.

[43] Parsons TA. The snapping scapula and subscapular exostoses. *J Bone Joint Surg Br.* 1973;55:345-349.

[44] de Haart M, van der Linden ES, de Vet HC, Arens H, Snoep G. The value of computed tomography in the diagnosis of grating scapula. *Skeletal Radiol.* 1994;23(5):357-359.

[45] Sans N, Jarlaud T, Sarrouy P, Giobbini K, Bellumore Y, Railhac JJ. [Snapping scapula: the value of 3D imaging]. *J Radiol.* 1999;80(4):379-381.

[46] Park JY, Hwang JT, Kim KM, Makkar D, Moon SG, Han KJ. How to assess scapular dyskinesis precisely: 3-dimensional wing computer tomography. A new diagnostic modality. *J Shoulder Elbow Surg.* 2013;22(8):1084-1091.

[47] E. G. McNally & J. L. Rees. Imaging in shoulder disorders. *Skeletal Radiol* (2007).

[48] Baker CL Jr, Liu SH: Neurovascular injuries to the shoulder. J Orthop Sport Phys Therapy 18:360-364, 1993.

[49] Masood Umer, Irfan Qadir, Mohsin Azam. Subacromial impingement syndrome. *Orthopedic Reviews* 2012; 4:e18.

[50] Higuchi T, Ogose A, Hotta T, et al. Clinical and imaging features of distended scapulothoracic bursitis: spontaneously regressed pseudotumoral lesion. *J Comput Assist Tomogr.* 2004;28(2):223-228.

[51] Ken O, Hatori M, Kokubun S. The MRI features and treatment of scapulothoracic bursitis: report of four cases. *Ups J Med Sci.* 2004;109(1):57-64.

[52] Chen CK, Wu HT, Chiou HJ, et al. Differentiating benign and malignant soft tissue masses by magnetic resonance imaging: role of tissue component analysis. *J Chin Med Assoc.* 2009;72(4):194-201.

[53] Datir A, James SL, Ali K, Lee J, Ahmad M, Saifuddin A. MRI of soft-tissue masses: the relationship between lesion size, depth, and diag nosis. *Clin Radiol.* 2008;63(4):373-378.

[54] Pang KK, Hughes T. MR imaging of the musculoskeletal soft tissue mass: is heterogeneity a sign of malignancy? *J Chin Med Assoc.* 2003;66(11):655-661.

[55] van Holsbeeck M, Strouse PJ. Sonography of the shoulder: evaluation of the subacromial-subdeltoid bursa. *AJR Am J Roentgenol* 1993; 160:561–564 .

[56] O'Connor PJ, Rankine J, Gibbon WW. Interobserver variation in sonography of the painful shoulder. *J Clin Ultrasound* 2005; 33: 53-56.

[57] Needell SD, Zlatkin MB, Sher JS, et al. MR. Imaging of rotator cuff: peritendinous and bone abnormalities in an asymptomatic population. AJR Am J Roentgenol 1996; 166: 863-870.

[58] MS Awerbuch. The clinical utility of ultrasonography for rotator cuff disease, shoulder impingement syndrome and subacromial bursitis. *Med J Aust* 2008; 188 (1): 50-53.

[59] Naranjo A, Marrerro-Pulido T, Ojeda S, et al. Abnormal sonographic findings in the asymptomatic arthritic shoulder. *Scand J Rheumatol* 2002; 31: 17-21.

[60] Zanetti M, Jost B, Hodler J, et al. MR imaging after rotator cuff repair: full thickness defects and bursitis-like subacromial abnormalities in asympto- matic subjects. *Skeletal Radiol* 2000; 29: 314-319.

[61] Huang CC, Ko SF, Ng SH, et al. Scapulothoracic bursitis of the chest wall: sonographic features with pathologic correlation. *J Ultrasound Med.* 2005;24(10):1437-1440.

[62] Naredo E, Möller I, Moragues C, et al. Interobserver reliability in musculoskeletal ultrasonography: results from a "Teach the Teachers" rheumatologist course. *Ann Rheum Dis* 2006; 65: 14-19.

[63] Saboeiro GR, Sofka CM. Imaging-guided treatment of scapulothoracic bursitis. *HSS J.* 2007;3(2):213-215.

[64] Michener LA, Walsworth MK, Burnet EN. Effectiveness of rehabilitation for patients with subacromial impingement syndrome: a systematic review. *J Hand Ther.* 2004 Apr-Jun;17(2):152-64.

[65] Morrison DS, Frogameni AD, Woodworth P. Non-operative treatment of subacromial impingement syndrome. *J Bone Joint Surg Am.* 1997 May;79(5):732-7.

[66] Chen MJL, Lew HL, Hsu TC, Tsai WC, Lin WC, Tang SFT, Lee YC, Hsu RCH, Chen CPC: Ultrasound-guided shoulder injections in the treatment of subacromial bursitis. *Am J Phys Med Rehabil* 2006; 85:31–35

[67] L. Mattei, M. Assom, M. Calò, F. Caranzan, R. Rossi, F. Castoldi, D. Blonna. Sicurezza Ed Efficacia Del Trattamento Del Dolore Di Spalla Mediante Infiltrazione Subacromiale Con Corticosteroidi In Pazienti Diabetici. *Poster session* SICSeG 2014

[68] Stitik TP, Foye PM, Fossati J. Shoulder injections for osteoarthritis and other disorders. *Phys Med Rehabil Clin N Am.* 2004 May;15(2):407-46.

[69] Gebremariam L, Hay EM, Koes BW, Huisstede BM. Effectiveness of surgical and postsurgical interventions for the subacromial impingement

syndrome: a systematic review. *Arch Phys Med Rehabil.* 2011 Nov;92(11):1900-13

[70] Magaji SA, Singh HP, Pandey RK. Arthroscopic subacromial decompression is effective in selected patients with shoulder impingement syndrome *J Bone Joint Surg Br.* 2012 Aug;94(8):1086-9.

[71] Checroun AJ, Dennis MG, Zuckerman JD. Open versus arthroscopic decompression for subacromial impingement. A comprehensive review of the literature from the last 25 years. *Bull Hosp Jt Dis.* 1998;57(3): 145-51.

[72] Ellman H. Shoulder arthroscopy: current indications and techniques. *Orthopedics.* 1988 Jan;11(1):45-51.

[73] Bigliani LU, Flatow EL, Deliz ED. College of Physicians and Surgeons, Columbia University, New York, NY. *Orthopaedic Review* [1991, 20(9):743-751]

[74] Donigan JA, Wolf BR. Arthroscopic subacromial decompression: acromioplasty versus bursectomy alone--does it really matter *Iowa Orthop J.* 2011;31:121-6. Review.

[75] Brislin KJ, Field LD, Savoie FH 3rd. Complications after arthroscopic rotator cuff repair. *Arthroscopy.* 2007 Feb;23(2):124-8.

[76] Manske RC, Reiman MP, Stovak ML. Nonoperative and operative management of snapping scapula. *Am J Sports Med.*

[77] Merolla G, Cerciello S, Paladini P, Porcellini G. Snapping scapula *Muscles Ligaments Tendons J.* 2013 Jul 9;3(2):80-90.

In: Bursitis of Major Joints
Editor: Alessandro Aprato

ISBN: 978-1-63482-295-4

Chapter II

Bursitis of the Elbow

Caterina Alluto*[*1], MD and Gabriele Agati[2], MD
[1] Department of Orthopaedics and Traumatology,
Ospedale Civile "E. Agnelli" of Pinerolo, Italy
[2] University of Torino, Department of Orthopaedics and Traumatology,
San Luigi Gonzaga Hospital of Orbassano, Torino, Italy

Abstract

Elbow bursitis can be classified in acute or chronic, septic or non septic and, according to the location, in superficial or deep. The two main bursae of the elbow are the olecranon bursa and the bicipitoradial bursa.

The olecranon bursa is situated between the olecranon process of the ulna, the triceps tendon and the overlying skin. Its superficial position and its poor vascularity make it vulnerable to inflammation, trauma and bacteria penetration. The bicipitoradial bursa is located between the radial tuberosity and the distal tendon of the biceps brachii and its function is to allow frictionless motion between these two structures during pronation and supination of the forearm. While the olecranon bursitis is a common condition, the bicipitoradial bursitis is quite rare. Trauma, overuse, crystal precipitation and rheumatoid arthritis are considered common causes.

* Corresponding author: Caterina Alluto, MD; Mail:Via Brigata Cagliari, 39, Pinerolo TO, Italy; Email: cate_alluto@hotmail.com.

The diagnosis of olecranon bursitis is usually clinical and the nodal point is to distinguish between septic and non septic bursitis to establish the right therapy.

The first approach consists in conservative treatment. If symptoms persist, bursal aspiration and corticosteroid injection are indicated.

Surgical treatment is performed in bursitis not responding to conservative therapy, chronic recurrent infection, resistant microorganism infection, foreign bodies or nerve compression at the cubital fossa.

Keywords: Olecranon bursitis, bicipitoradial bursitis, distal biceps tendon

Introduction

The main bursa of the elbow is the olecranon one; its superficial position and its poor vascularity make it vulnerable to inflammation, trauma and bacteria penetration wherein the bursal cavity becomes inflamed and its volume is significantly increased. It is more frequent in male aged 30 to 60 but its real incidence is not known, because most of them are treated conservatively and do not require hospital admission. It can be caused by different conditions, such as direct trauma, repetitive trauma, systemic inflammatory diseases or infection. In addition to the olecranon bursa, the elbow joint presents some other bursae (superficial or deep), which presence can be variable. The main deep bursae are located in the cubital fossa and they are the bicipitoradial bursa and the interosseous bursa. The bicipitoradial bursa lies between the distal biceps tendon and the radial tuberosity and it allows frictionless motion between these structures during pronation and supination.

The bicipitoradial bursitis is a rare condition caused by repetitive mechanical trauma, synovitis, rheumatic diseases or partial tear of the biceps tendon. Few cases are reported in literature but it should be considered as a possible cause of anterior forearm pain. The diagnosis of bicipitoradial bursitis requires instead imaging support such as US or MRI and a differential diagnosis with tenosynovitis, cysts, lipoma or malignant tumors.

Anatomy

The elbow is a complex joint composed by three bones, the humerus, the ulna and the radius. The humeroulnar joint allows flexion and extension of the elbow. The humeroradial joint and the proximal radioulnar joints are involved in prono-supination movements and work in coordination with the distal radioulnar joint. The extension of the elbow is due to two muscles, the triceps brachii and anconeus.

The triceps brachii is a long and powerful muscle that forms all the posterior musculature of the arm. Two humeral heads and one scapular head that join in a common large tendon and insert into the olecranon process of the ulna compose it. The anconeus is a small muscle that originates in the lateral epicondyle and ends at the dorsal lateral surface of the proximal ulna. The superficial anconeus fascia is continuous with the lateral triceps tendon, forming a common insertion on the lateral surface of the ulna and the deep fascia of the forearm. [1]

The flexor group includes the biceps brachii, the brachialis and the brachioradialis.

The biceps brachii and the brachialis run on the anterior surface of the arm and they are considered the main elbow flexors. The biceps brachii, composed by the long and the short heads, ends with a narrow tendon on the posterior edge of radial tuberosity. When the forearm is pronated, biceps works as a powerful supinator. Deep to the biceps there is the brachialis muscle that is a pure flexor. It originates with a large insertion from the anterior surface of the humerus and it ends on the tuberosity of the ulna at the base of the coronoid process. The brachioradialis is the third flexor muscle of the elbow, running from the distal end of the humerus to the radial styolid process.

Since the 18th century several authors have described different number of elbow bursae [2-4] They consist in closed sacs, lined by synovial cells, situated around the joint and tendon insertions and their function is to reduce the friction between connective tissue structures involved in joint motion. They can be divided into superficial, in the subcutaneous tissue, and deep, between muscles and bone tissue.

In the posterior elbow is well known the olecranon bursa, a superficial structure situated between the olecranon process of the ulna, the triceps tendon and the overlying skin. It is not present in child under the age of 7 years and its size increases with age. [5] A deep intra-tendinous bursa is frequently located inside the triceps tendon fibers at their insertion on the olecranon process and another little deep bursa can be found between the tendon and the tip of the olecranon (sub-tendineous borsa). Two superficial bursae can be occasionally located above the epicondyle or, more frequently, on the epitroclea.

The main deep bursa of the elbow is the bicipitoradial bursa, located between the radial tuberosity anteriorly and the distal tendon of the biceps brachii posteriorly and its function is to allow frictionless motion between these two structures during pronation and supination of the forearm. [6] Its size has been evaluated between 2,4 cm and 3,9 cm. It sometimes presents internal septation [7] and a possible communication with the joint cavity is controversial. [8,9] When the forearm is supinated the bicipitoradial bursa surrounds the distal biceps tendon; during pronation the radius rotates posteriorly and the bursa is compressed between the tendon and the radial tuberosity. An interosseus ulnar bursa that lies between the biceps tendon, the ulna and the muscles above the radius was also observed. The bicipitoradial bursa can be in communication with this bursa.

Physiopathology

Bursitis are a common cause of musculoskeletal pain. They can be classified in acute or chronic, septic or non septic and, according to the location, in superficial or deep. Aseptic bursitis can be further classified in traumatic, idiopathic or crystal-induced.

Olecranon bursitis is the most common form of elbow bursitis; the quite superficial position of this bursa make it vulnerable to trauma and penetrating injuries.

The acute form is frequently caused by direct trauma on the elbow, sport injuries or falling on the olecranon process. Trauma causes an acute local inflammatory response and resulting iperproduction of synovial fluid and bursal swelling. Persisting of the inflammation may results into permanent damage of the bursal epithelial layer. If elongated by fluid, the bursa may break into the subcutaneous tissue of the forearm.

Chronic inflammation of this bursa is frequently the result of overuse or repetitive trauma as in certain occupational diseases (gardeners, miners, carpenters), in students or athletes (volleyball, ice hockey, football). For this reason it is also known as "student's elbow" or "miner's elbow". [10]

Olecranon bursitis may also be related to systemic inflammatory diseases such as rheumatoid arthritis, [11] condrocalcinosis, uremia or gout that causes crystal precipitation within the bursa. [12] Obesity, diabetes mellitus and inflammatory arthropathies are considered risk factors.

Acute gouty bursitis is mainly due to the precipitation of monosodium urate crystals into the bursal sac; the urate concentration can increase also during the resorption of traumatic swelling. The bursal walls become thicker, poorly delimited from the surrounding tissues and the cavity is filled with proliferated synovia. Canoso reported a series of 15 patients and 40% of them presented concomitant acute gouty arthritis of another joint, but the involvement of the adjacent joint has not been related. [13] Some authors described multiple rice body formation in association with rheumatoid arthritis, [14] tuberculous or nonspecific bursitis. [15, 16] Olecranon bursitis has been observed in hemodialysis patients, also known as "dialysis elbow", and it usually develops at the same side of the arteriovenous fistula. [17] The causes of this phenomenon are still unknown; mechanical factors due to patients' position on their elbow during the therapy, uremic serositis and anticoagulant therapy have been suggested. [18, 19]

Septic bursitis represent approximately one third of all olecranon bursitis, most often caused by bacterial agents. [20] Infection may be due to skin lesions, secondary spread after previous non septic bursitis or direct transcutaneous penetration. Preexisting bursal disease (gout or rheumatoid arthritis) and previous aspiration or infiltration of the bursa can facilitate the onset of a septic bursitis. Hematogenous seeding is rare, probably for the poor vascularization of the bursal fluid.

Immunodeficiency, chronic alcohol abuse, systemic steroid therapy, chronic obstructive pulmonary disease and chronic renal failure are considered systemic risk factors. Furthermore prior history of septic bursitis increases the risk of bursal infection.

Usually septic bursitis does not hesitate in joint infection. This may occurs after surgical approach to the elbow or in extended contaminated wounds.

Staphylococcus Aureus and group A beta-hemolytic Streptococcus are the most common infective agents, causing from 80% to 100% of septic bursitis. [10, 21] A small percentage is due to Staphylococcus epidermidis, whereas Gram-negative infections are rare. Tuberoculous infection was common in the preantibiotic era; some cases of nontuberculous mycobacteria infection have been described, especially in immune-compromise patients. [22]

Bicipitoradial bursitis (BRB) is a rare condition. The main etiologic factor is repetitive pronation and supination movements of the elbow; it has been described in association with tendinosis, partial or complete tear of the distal biceps tendon. [23] Williams et al. reported an incidence of 55% of BRB in association with partial tear of the biceps tendon. [24] Other causes may be synovial chondromatosis, capsular synovial cyst, bone proliferation, rheumatological diseases or infection. [6, 25] During pronation the bursa is compressed between the tendon and the radial tuberosity; if the bursa is rather enlarged, it can cause a compression of the radial nerve; [26, 27] with an important distension of the bursa or with a communication between the BRB and the interosseous bursa also the median nerve may be compressed. [8]

Infection of this deep bursa is rare.

Clinical Evaluation

The diagnosis of olecranon bursitis is usually clinical.

Physical examination reveals swelling, tenderness over the tip of the olecranon, redness, and local inflammatory reaction (Figure 1). Bursitis are often painless and joint motion is usually preserved. In acute forms extensive peribursal cellulitis may be observed. In chronic patients bursal consistency is more solid and small lumps can be palpated. When symptomatic, bursitis may cause pain with elbow flexion more than 90 degrees, because the intrabursal pressure increases between 60 and 90 degrees and it decreases in extension. In infections fever, pain and local warmth may be present. The risk of septic bursitis is increased in case of skin lesions as wounds or abrasions. About one third of cases of septic bursitis report a history of previous aseptic olecranon bursitis; this can be explained by the reduced capacity of the bursa, previously damaged by inflammatory processes, to prevent bacteria penetration.

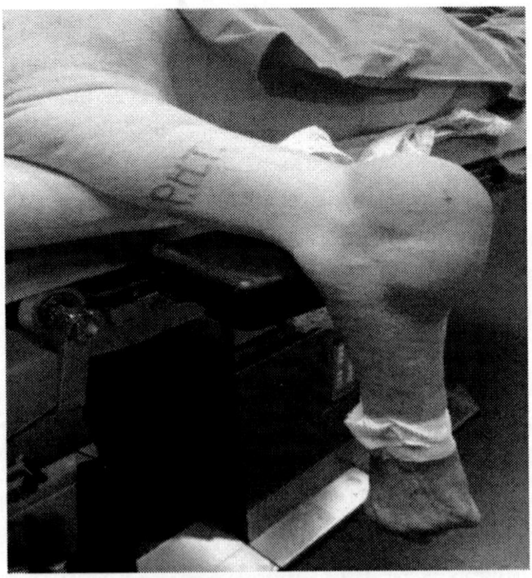

a

Figure 1. (Continued).

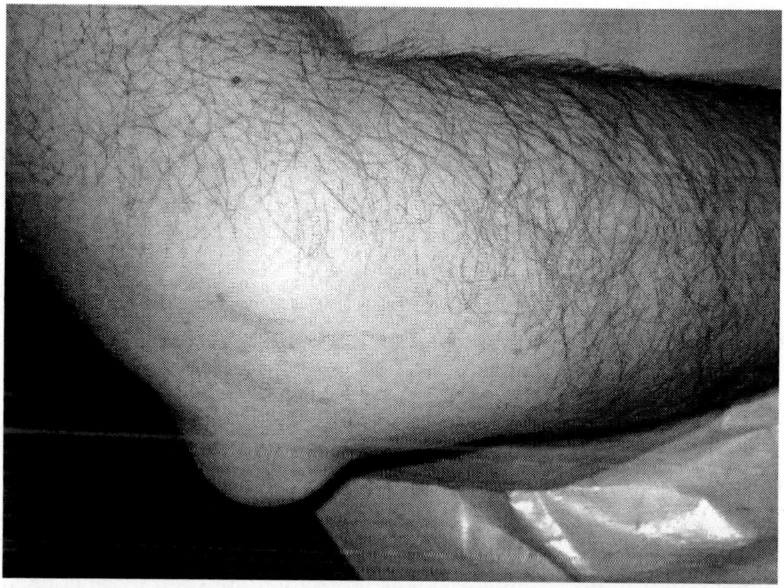

b

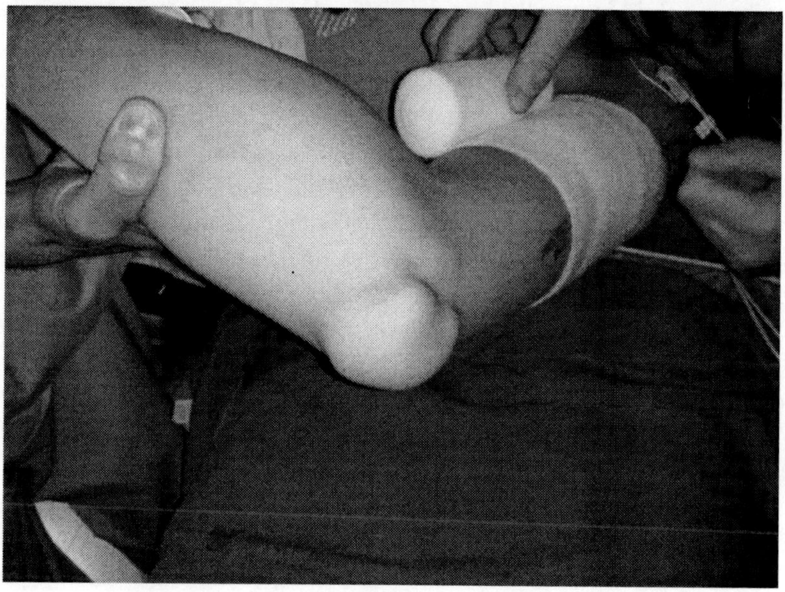

c

Figure 1. (a, b, c). Clinical presentation of olecranon bursitis.

In patients affected by rheumatoid arthritis, the bursa can dissect and originate a swelling within the triceps or it can communicate with the joint cavity and spread anteriorly in the forearm. [28]

The clinical differentiation between septic or non-septic bursitis is difficult because of the lack of specific signs and symptoms. The diagnosis of infection requires the aspiration of the bursal fluid, essential also to direct specific therapy. This test can be considered as highly sensitive and specific, but false-positive cultures can be due to contamination from skin surface or non-sterile procedure. The macroscopic characteristics of the fluid give a first diagnostic hypothesis: while a clear, serous or hemorrhagic aspirate suggests non septic bursitis, purulent fluid hints for infection, but also in rheumatoid or gouty bursitis it may be rather turbid. Hemorrhagic bursitis occurs in 21% of cases of traumatic bursitis, in 9% of septic bursitis and in 13% of rheumatoid bursitis. In microscopic analysis cell count, glucose concentration, Gram's stain, crystal examination and culture with sensitivity test are recommended. [12,29] In septic bursitis white cell count is usually greater than 3000 μ/L with percentage of polymorphonuclear cells more than 50%. Glucose concentration of the bursal fluid is usually less than 50% of the serum concentration and its absolute value is lower than 31 mg/dl, but the importance of these data to distinguish between septic and aseptic bursitis is not established. [30] Furthermore, Gram's stain is negative in 30% of septic bursitis and this result cannot exclude an infection. In aspirate examination of gouty bursitis monosodium urate crystals are visible by polarized light microscopy and a relatively low white blood cells and percentage of polymorphonuclear cells was observed compared with articular gout. [13] The presence of calcium pyrophosphate dihydrate is typical of pseudogout.

If there is a suspicion of articular infection, the joint must be aspirated and the synovial fluid analyzed. The aspiration must be performed in sterile condition and through uninjured skin.

Bicipitoradial bursitis clinically presents as a mass in the anterior surface of the proximal forearm; pain and impairment of range of motion are common symptoms, especially in pronation when the bursa is compressed between radius and biceps insertion. In association with tendinosis of the distal biceps tendon, pronation and elbow flection can also be painful. When the bursa is quite enlarged, it can have a mass effect on the cubital fossa resulting in compression of the radial nerve or the medial nerve. Symptoms depend on which branch is involved: compression of superficial branch of radial nerve originates just sensitive symptoms at the dorsum of the hand and fingers, while compression of the posterior interosseous nerve leads to weakness of the extensor muscles of the forearm.

Imaging

Although the diagnosis of olecranon bursitis is mainly clinical, conventional radiographs are useful to exclude fracture of the olecranon if there is a history of trauma or osteomyelitis is suspected. In several non traumatic bursitis, calcifications of the triceps tendon insertion, spur or prominence of the olecranon process may be observed (Figure 2).

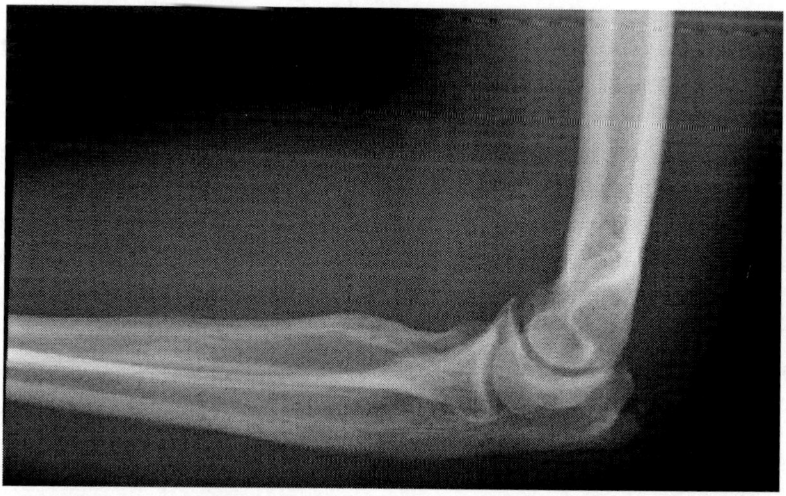

Figure 2. Typical spur of the olecranon in recurrent aseptic olecranon bursitis (lateral X-rays view).

Ultrasound helps to establish bursal content and characteristics of the fluid and can identify rheumatoid nodules or gouty tophi as hyperechoic spots. [31]

Magnetic resonance imaging can be indicated in septic bursitis to evaluate abscess formation or concomitant osteomyelitis. The bursa appears with a hypo-intensity signal on T1-weighted sequences and variable intensity on T2-weighted images; swelling and edema of the surrounding soft tissues can be showed. Lobulation, complexity of the bursal fluid, and thickening of the triceps tendon result more accentuated in septic bursitis compared with non septic ones. [32]

In rare cases rice body formation was observed, especially in association with rheumatoid arthritis. [16]

The diagnosis of bicipitoradial bursitis is more supported by imaging studies. In normal condition, the bursa is not visible neither on ultrasound, nor on magnetic resonance imaging; it become apparent in case of inflammation and enlargement. [27,33]

Standard X-Rays can identify small calcifications on the biceps tendon or roughness of the radial tuberosity, but these findings can be occasional and cannot be considered diagnostic signs.

Ultrasound is a cheap and easy technique allowing identification of the distended bursa surrounding the distal biceps tendon. The bursa appears as an anechoic formation with internal septa between the biceps tendon and the radial tuberosity, better visualized if the forearm is pronated. Increased vascularity may be noted at color Doppler imaging. [34,35] US can also provide information about macroscopic radial nerve damage or compression; [7] aspiration and intrabursal injections of steroids can be performed at the same time as the diagnostic examination, avoinding the risk of damage neurovascular structures.

Magnetic resonance imaging allow a more accurate diagnosis of BRB, its relationship with the distal biceps tendon and its effect on the radial nerve. The posterior wall of the bursa is well visualized near to the radial cortex, but the anterior wall is difficult to recognize from the paratenon of the biceps tendon. When the bursa is much enlarged, it is hard to distinguish a bicipitoradial bursitis from an interosseous bursitis. [8]

The signal intensity characteristics suggest the nature of the bursal fluid. On T2- weighted images the bursa appears as a homogeneous increased intensity area compared with fat intensity; hypointense septa may be identified.

Differential diagnosis of BRB includes lipoma of the cubital region, lipoma arborescens, infections, tenosynovitis, ganglion cysts, pigmented villonodular synovitis or synovial chondromatosis and malignant tumors. [36-38]

In claustrophobic patients, pacemaker or other contraindications to MRI, contrast-enhanced CT may be performed. It shows the bursitis as fusiform sac with uniform density and it can also evaluate integrity of the biceps tendon or hyperostosis of the radius.

In few cases CT or RM imaging cannot differentiate bursitis from a neoplasm and the true diagnosis can be reached only with an histological examination.

Conservative Treatment

Treatment of acute olecranon bursitis consists in an initially conservative approach based on local ice application, rest and NSAIDs. If symptoms do not regress, aspiration of bursal fluid and corticosteroid injection are indicated, followed by compressive elastic bandage. The aspiration should be performed in aseptic setting using an 18 or 20 gauge needle. The penetration of the needle in the medial side of the elbow should be avoided for the risk of ulnar nerve damage and the elbow capsule should not be violated to prevent secondary iatrogenic septic arthritis.

Weinstein et al. demonstrated better results in patients treated by aspiration associated with steroid injection compared with those treated by aspiration alone. [39] The main complication of local corticosteroid therapy is skin atrophy and pain is frequent after the injection, as a possible expression of subclinical atrophy. The use of topic steroid is associated with an increased risk of septic bursitis, also with low-dose administration. [39]

Septic bursitis treatment requires prompt empiric antibiotic therapy with penicillase-resistant penicillin, such as oxacillin. Later the therapy is modified depending on culture examination results and bursal drainage with specific antbiotic; lavage with sterile saline solution through a large needle can improve the evacuation.

Oral administration of oxacillin and penicillin has been shown to allow reaching of bactericidal concentration in bursal fluid. [40] In case of systemic symptoms, fever or cellulitis parenteral treatment is indicated. The duration of the therapy depends on clinical evolution, comorbidities and the time between symptoms appearance and therapy beginning. Ho and Su recommended 5 days of therapy after sterile aspiration of the bursa. [40] Roschmann and Bell reported that immunocompromised patients required a mean of 11 days of antibiotic treatment to obtain negative culture. [41]

Previous infection of the same bursa or preexisting bursal diseases such as tophaceous gout or rheumatoid nodule may reduce the efficacy of drainage and antibiotic therapy.

In bicipitoradial bursitis therapeutic aspiration and corticosteroid injection can be performed at the same time as the sonography examination, as previously described.

Surgical Treatment

Surgical treatment of olecranon bursitis is indicated in patients not responding to conservative treatment, in chronic recurring infection, in septic bursitis after previous surgical treatment, in resistant microorganism infection and in case of extended infection or foreign body. [42]

Standard open bursectomy or endoscopic resection can be carried out.

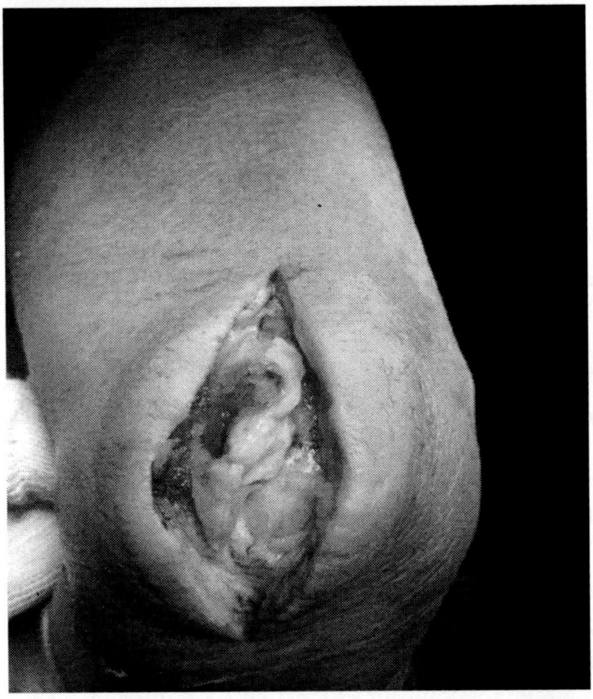

Figure 3. Intraoperative image showing macroscopic aspect of septic olecranon bursitis.

Open bursectomy is performed through a straight posterior or postero-lateral approach to avoid the incision being directly over the tip of the olecranon. The use of a tourniquet is suggested. The bursa should be isolated and removed as a single structure to ensure complete excision of all bursal tissue (Figures 3,4,5). A spur on the olecranon process, if present, should be removed (Figure 6). Meticulous closure of the subcutaneous tissues with absorbable suture followed by compressive bandage avoid the formation of a dead space and reduce the risk of relapse. The main complication of open olecranon bursectomy is the wound no-healing. Some authors reported problematic wounds in more than 25% of patients, such as persisting exudation and in some cases skin necrosis requiring flap surgery. [43] Postoperatively immobilization with a splint for 2 weeks is recommended to prevent wound complications.

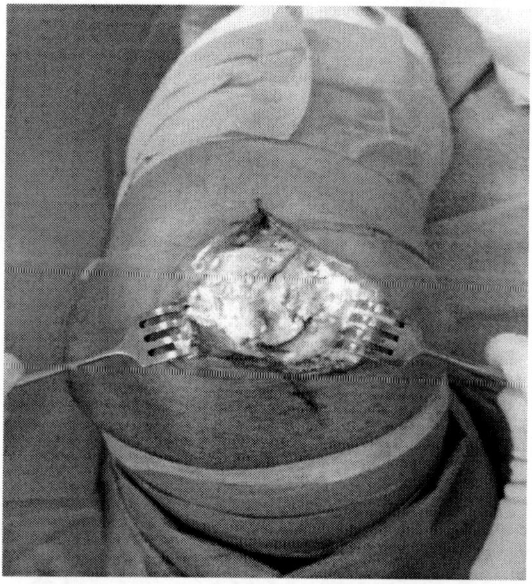

a

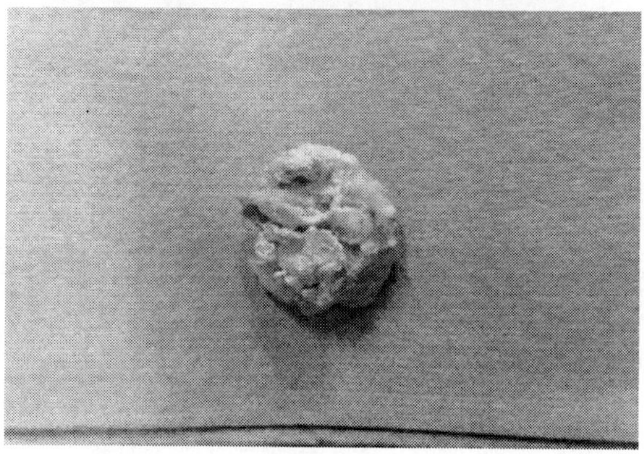

b

Figure 4. a) Intraoperative aspect of olecranon bursitis in rheumatoid arthritis patient. b) bursal tissue after surgical excision.

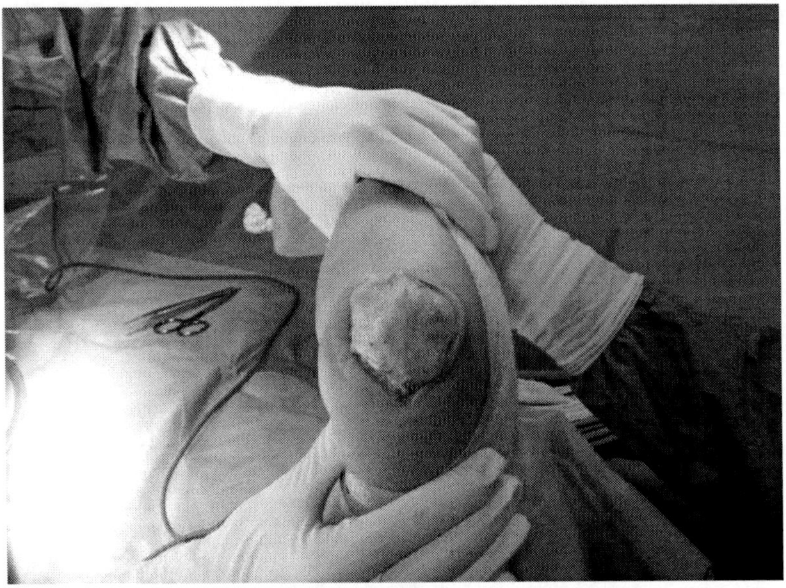

a

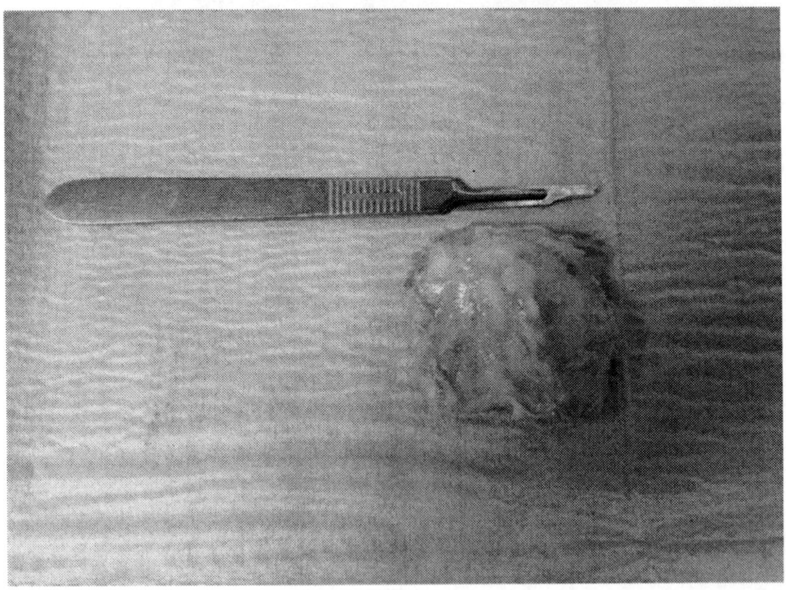

b

Figure 5. a) Intraoperative aspect of chronic aseptic olecranon bursitis. b) bursal tissue after surgical excision.

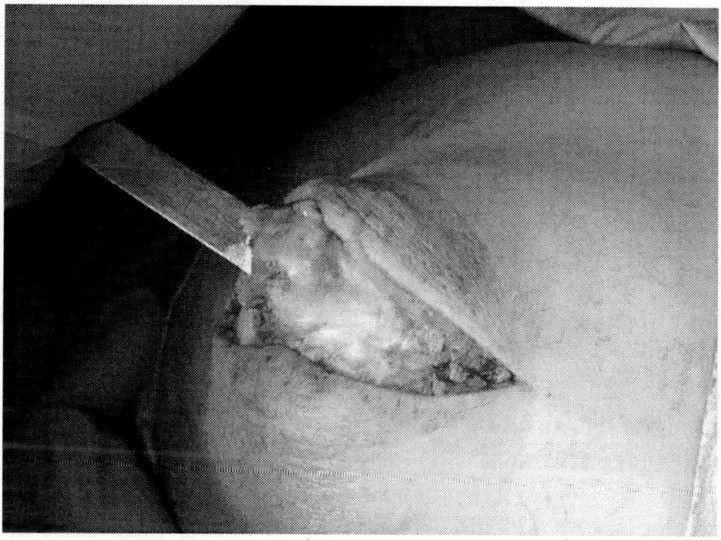

Figure 6. Intraoperative image showing removal of olecranon spur.

Stewart el al. reported 60% rate of recurrence or symptoms persistence in patients affected by rheumatoid arthritis; [44] in these cases surgical indication must be carefully evaluated.

More recently endoscopic technique has been described. [45,46] The patient can be placed in supine position or lateral decubitus. The skin portals should be made 1 cm away from the bursal edge. The bursa is previously inflated with saline solution to better identify bursal walls. The bursa can be excised with an inside-out technique, removing first the subcutaneous tissue and then the deep portion. Care must be taken to avoid skin penetration and ulnar nerve damage. The advantages of the endoscopic technique compared with the open surgery are faster healing times and avoiding a scare over the olecranon, which can become painful. Complications of endoscopy include hematoma and persistent sinus from skin perforation. Tu et al. proposed an extrabursal excision technique in aseptic bursitis, reporting a lower rate of skin perforation. [47]

The surgical treatment of the bicipitoradial bursitis is indicated in case of recurrence of swelling and pain after conservative treatment, in infection, in presence of nerve compression and neurological impairment and in biceps tendon degeneration. [33] An antero-lateral incision is usually performed, with patient in supine position. The posterior interosseous nerve must be identified at the lateral margin of the brachialis muscle and protected. The bursa and the radial tuberosity are exposed after splitting of the supinator muscle. In case of capsular tear, it should be repaired to avoid a new formation of synovial cist. Partial tear or degeneration of the biceps tendon can be treated simultaneously.

Conclusion

The olecranon bursitis is a common disease, with different etiological factors: direct trauma, overuse, chronic inflammatory diseases or infection.

The distinction between septic and aseptic bursitis is the most important step to set the correct therapy. Septic bursitis rarely presents with specific clinical signs and the diagnosis always requires the aspiration and the examination of the bursal fluid.

The first approach to aseptic olecranon bursitis is always conservative and consists of rest, ice, NSAIDs, bursal fluid aspiration and local corticosteroid injection. In case of infection, a correct antibiotic therapy based on the fluid examination may be administered. The surgical treatment is indicated in bursitis not responding to conservative treatment. It is important to remove the bursa as an intact structure to be sure of the complete excision of the bursal tissue. Although arthroscopic techniques have been described for the olecranon bursectomy, most of surgeons prefer an open approach, easier and quicker.

The bicipitoradial bursitis is instead a rare condition, which should be considered as a possible cause of anterior forearm pain and compression of the radial nerve. The diagnosis can in fact be difficult and it always requires imaging support such as RMI or US. Surgical treatment is indicated for recurrent bursitis, nerve compression or infection.

References

[1] Keener JD, Chafik D, Kim HM, Galatz LM, Yamaguchi K. Insertional anatomy of the triceps brachii tendon. *J Shoulder Elbow Srg.* 2010;19:399-405.

[2] Monro A. A description of all the Bursae Mucosae of the Human Body. London, 1788.

[3] Schreger BG. De bursis mucosis subcutaneis. *Enlargen* 1825, plate VII.

[4] Canoso JJ. Bursae, tendons and ligaments. *Clin Rheum Dis.* 1981; 7:189-221.

[5] Chen J, Alk D, Eventov I, Wientroub S. Development of the olecranon bursa. An anatomic cadaver study. *Acta Orthop Scand.* 1987; 58:408-09.

[6] Matsumoto K, Hukuda S, Fujita M, Kakimoto A, Tachibana S. Cubital bursitis caused by localized synovial chondromatosis of the elbow. A Case Report. *J Bone Joint Surg Am.* 1996;78:275-7.

[7] Draghi F, Gregoli B, Sileo C. Sonography of the bicipitoradial bursa. A short pictorial essay. *J ultrasound.* 2012;15:39-41.

[8] Skaf AY, Boutin RD, Dantas RW, Hooper AW, Muhle C, Chou DS, Lektrakul N, Trudell DJ, Haghighi P, Resnick DL. Bicipitoradial bursitis: MR imaging findings in eight patients and anatomic data from contrast material opacification of bursae followed by routine radiography and MR imaging in cadavers. Radiology. 1999;212:111-6.

[9] Chen WS, Wang CJ. Recalcitrant bicipital radial bursitis. *Arch Orthop Trauma Surg* 1999; 119:105-8.

[10] Ho G Jr, Tice AD, Kaplan SR. Septic bursitis in the prepatellar and olecranon bursae: an analysis of 25 cases. *Ann Intern Med* 1978;89:21–27.

[11] Macfarlane JD, van der Linden SJ. Leaking rheumatoid olecranon bursitis as a cause of forearm swelling. *Ann Rheum Dis.* 1981; 40:309-11.

[12] McAfee JH, Smith DL. Olecranon and prepatellar bursitis. Diagnosis and treatment. *West J Med.* 1988; 149:607-10.

[13] Canoso JJ, Yood RA. Acute gouty bursitis: report of 15 cases. *Ann Rheum Dis.* 1979; 38:326-8.

[14] Popert AJ, Scott DL, Wainwright AC, Walton KW, Williamson N, Chapman JH. Frequency of occurrence, mode of development, and significance or rice bodies in rheumatoid joints. *Ann Rheum Dis.* 1982; 41:109-17.

[15] Holder SF, Hopson CN, Vonkuster LC. Tuberculous arthritis of the elbow presenting as chronic bursitis of the olecranon. A case report. *J Bone Joint Surg Am,* 1985; 67:1127-1129.

[16] Matsumoto T, Fujita K, Fujioka H, Matsushima S, Kouso K, Yamaguchi S, Kurosaka M, Yoshiya S. Massive nonspecific olecranon bursitis with multiple rice bodies. *J Shoulder Elbow Surg.* 2004; 13:680-3.

[17] Jain VK, Cestero RV, Baum J. Septic and aseptic olecranon bursitis in patients on maintenance hemodialysis. *Clin Exp Dial Apheresis.* 1981; 5:405-14.

[18] Senecal 1, Leblanc M. Olecranon bursitis in chronic haemodialysis patients. *Nephrol Dial Transpl* 2001; 16:1956–7.

[19] Chao CT, Wu MS. Dialysis elbow. *QJM.* 2012; 105:485-6.
[20] Stell IM. Septic and non-septic olecranon bursitis in the accident and emergency department-an approach to management. *J Accid Emerg Med* 1996; 13:351-353.
[21] Ziimermann B III, Mikolich DJ, HO Jr G. Septic bursitis. *Semin Arthritis Rheum* 1995; 24:391-410.
[22] Garrigues GE, Aldridge JM 3rd, Toth AP, Stout JE. Nontuberculous mycobacterial olecranon bursitis: case reports and literature review. *J Shoulder Elbow Surg.* 2009; 18:e1-5.
[23] Karanjia ND, Stiles PJ. Cubital bursitis. *J Bone Joint Sung* [Br] 1988; 70: 832-33.
[24] Williams BD, Schweitzer ME, Weishaupt D, Lerman J, Rubenstein DL, Miller LS, Rosenberg ZS. Partial tears of the distal biceps tendon: MR appearance and associated clinical findings. *Skeletal Radiol.* 2001; 30:560-4.
[25] Rasing LA, van Kampen A. A rare case of enthesopathy of the bicipital tuberositas of the radius. *Arch Orthop Trauma Surg.* 2000; 120:601-2.
[26] Ferdinand BD, Rosenberg ZS, Schweitzer ME, Stuchin SA, Jazrawi LM, Lenzo SR, Meislin RJ, Kiprovski K. MR imaging features of radial tunnel syndrome: initial experience. *Radiology.* 2006; 240:161-8.
[27] Espiga X, Alentorn-Geli E, Lozano C, Cebamanos J. Symptomatic bicipitoradial bursitis: a report of two cases and review of the literature. *J Shoulder Elbow Surg.* 2011; 20:e5-9.
[28] Petrie JP, Wigley RD. Proximal dissection of the olecranon bursa in rheumatoid arthritis. *Rheumatol Int.* 1984; 4:139-40.
[29] Shell D, Perkins R, Cosgarea A. Septic olecranon bursitis: recognition and treatment. *J Am Board Fam Pract.* 1995; 8:217-20.
[30] Baumbach SF, Lobo CM, Badyine I, Mutschler W, Kanz KG. Prepatellar and olecranon bursitis: literature review and development of a treatment algorithm. *Arch Orthop Trauma Surg.* 2014; 134:359-70.
[31] Radunovic G, Vlad V, Micu MC, Nestorova R, Petranova T, Porta F, Iagnocco A. Ultrasound assessment of the elbow. *Med Ultrason.* 2012; 14:141-6.
[32] Floemer F, Morrison WB, Bongartz G, Ledermann HP. MRI characteristics of olecranon bursitis. *AJR Am J Roentgenol.* 2004; 183:29-34.
[33] Choi TL, Lui TH. Bicipitoradial Bursitis: a review of clinical presentation and treatment. *Journal of Orthopaedics, Trauma and Rehabilitation.* 2014;18:7 – 11.

[34] Liessi G, Cesari S, Spaliviero B, Dell'Antonio C, Avventi P. The US, CT and MR findings of cubital bursitis: a report of five cases. *Skeletal Radiol.* 1996; 25:471-5.

[35] Sofka CM, Adler RS. Sonography of cubital bursitis. *AJR Am J Roentgenol.* 2004; 183:51-3.

[36] Valbuena SE, O'Toole GA, Roulot E. Compression of the median nerve in the proximal forearm by a giant lipoma: A case report. *J Brachial Plex Peripher Nerve Inj.* 2008; 10:3-17.

[37] Dinauer P, Bojescul JA, Kaplan KJ, Litts C. Bilateral lipoma arborescens of the bicipitoradial bursa. Skeletal Radiol. 2002; 31:661-5.

[38] Singh AP, Chadha M, Singh AP, Mahajan S. Isolated tuberculous biceps tenosynovitis bicipitoradial bursitis: a case report. *J Shoulder Elbow Surg.* 2009; 18:e30-3.

[39] Weinstein PS, Canoso JJ, Wohlgethan JR. Long-term follow-up of corticosteroid injection for traumatic olecranon bursitis. *Ann Rheum Dis.* 1984; 43:44-6.

[40] Ho G Jr, Su EY. Antibiotic therapy of septic bursitis. Its implication in the treatment of septic arthritis. *Arthritis Rheum.* 1981; 24:905-11.

[41] Roschmann RA, Bell CL. Septic bursitis in immunocompromised patients. *Am J Med.* 1987; 83:661-5.

[42] Morrey BF. The elbow and its disorders. 3rd ed. 2000 Philadelphia: *WB Saunders.*

[43] Degreef I, De Smet L. Complications following resection of the olecranon bursa. *Acta Orthop Belg.* 2006; 72:400-3.

[44] Stewart NJ, Manzanares JB, Morrey BF. Surgical treatment of aseptic olecranon bursitis. *J Shoulder Elbow Surg.* 1997; 6:49-54.

[45] Kerr DR, Carpenter CW. Arthroscopic resection of olecranon and prepatellar bursae. *Arthroscopy.* 1990; 6:86-8.

[46] Ogilvie-Harris DJ, Gilbart M.Endoscopic bursal resection: the olecranon bursa and prepatellar bursa. *Arthroscopy.* 2000; 16:249-53.

[47] Tu CG, McGuire DT, Morse LP, Bain GI. Olecranon extrabursal endoscopic bursectomy. *Tech Hand Up Extrem Surg.* 2013; 17:173-5.

In: Bursitis of Major Joints
Editor: Alessandro Aprato
ISBN: 978-1-63482-295-4

Chapter III

Bursitis Around the Hip

Alessandro Aprato*, MD, Laura Ravera, MD,
Marco Maria Favuto, MD,
and Alessandro Masse', MD, Prof.
University of Torino, Department of Orthopaedics and Traumatology,
Ospedale San Luigi di Orbassano, Torino, Italy

Abstract

Hip bursitis is a frustrating condition encountered regularly by primary care physicians and orthopaedists. The causes of GTPS can be traumatic and nontraumatic. Risk factors are various and variously described, including age older than 40 years, female gender, ipsilateral ITB pain, knee osteoarthritis (OA), obesity, and low back pain (LBP).

In the literature there have been described more than 20 bursae in the trochanteric region. Three are certainly the most representative: the gluteus minimus bursa, the subgluteus maximus and subgluteus medius bursae.

Patients are suffering from pain radiating to the posterolateral aspect of the thigh, paraesthesiae in the legs, and tenderness over the iliotibial tract. Often the symptoms are mild, with the patient treating himself

* Corresponding author: Alessandro Aprato, MD; Viale 25 Aprile, 10133, Torino, Italy; Ph: (+39) 3386880640; Email: ale_aprato@hotmail.com.

successfully through activity modification and other conservative measures, including relative rest, ice, compression, elevation, anti-inflammatory medication and treatment modalities such as ultrasound and electrical stimulation, combined with a structured rehabilitation program. Patients whose symptoms persist despite conservative therapy are likely to benefit from an injection of corticosteroid and anaesthetic into the inflamed bursa. More invasive surgical interventions have been reported to provide pain relief when previous treatment modalities fail. In this chapter, we review the pathogenesis, common initial symptoms, diagnostic approach, and treatment options for trochanteric bursitis.

Keywords: Greater trochanteric pain syndrome, bursitis, low back pain, subgluteal bursae

Introduction

Hip bursitis is a frustrating condition encountered regularly by primary care physicians and orthopaedists. Evaluating these problems can be challenging because of the myriad of potential causes. Additionally the complex anatomy of the trochanteric bursae, associated myotendinous and fascial structures, and the etiologic factors contributing to pain have been described inconsistently.

Described for years as trochanteric bursitis, advanced imaging and surgical findings in patients with pain and tenderness of the greater trochanteric (GT) region, buttock and lateral thigh, have evidenced disorders involving incomplete tearing or avulsion of the anterior aspect of the gluteus medius and gluteus minimus tendons, external coxa saltans (snapping hip), and enthesiopathy, with no real bursal involvement [1-4].

In 1923, Stegemann [5] used the term “trochanteric bursitis” to describe chronic, recurrent lateral hip pain. Also called the “great mimicker”, it shared clinical features with other conditions that could be mistaken for other diagnoses. However the term “trochanteric bursitis” itself may be a misnomer, since three of Celsus’ cardinal signs of inflammation (redness, warmth, and swelling) are usually not seen [6]. In 1958, Leonard [7] called this condition “trochanteric syndrome”, reflecting the multitude of causes for pain localized to the “trochanter major”. More recently, the “greater trochanteric pain syndrome” (GTPS) [8] has been used with increasing frequency to describe pain and tenderness in the region of the greater trochanter and the juxtaposed soft tissues of the buttock and lateral proximal thigh.

GTPS is more frequent in women (F:M . 4:1) aged 40–60 years, and affects from 10 to 25% of the general population, and up to 35% in patients who have leg length discrepancies and low back pain [9-11]. Abnormal force vectors acting across the hip, leading to abnormal hip biomechanics, are predisposing factors, but, age, gender, ipsilateral iliotibial band pain, knee osteoarthritis, obesity, low back pain and specific sporting activities have to be considered as well [8,9,12-14].

The higher prevalence in women could be related to the configuration of their pelvis, whilst obesity results in low back pain and overloading of the hip and the knee [9]. Though common in sedentary patients, runners adducting the hips beyond midline are also particularly predisposed, and road runners, exposed to increased friction over the greater trochanter and the iliotibial tract during the flexion and extension of the hip, may develop GTPS of the 'downside leg' (the nearest to the road side) [15,16].

However, repetitive activity, acute trauma, crystal deposition, infection (especially tuberculosis), associated osteoarthritis, rheumatoid arthritis and lumbosacral disorders have to be excluded [17,18].

Anatomy

In the literature there have been described more than 20 bursae in the trochanteric region [19]. Three are certainly the most representative: the gluteus minimus bursa, the subgluteus maximus and subgluteus medius bursae.

Bursae are fluid-filled sacs that provide cushioning and a gliding interface between bony prominences and the surrounding soft tissues. Overlying the lateral aspect of the greater femoral trochanter, the trochanteric bursae are commonly implicated as a cause of lateral hip pain [20]. The anatomy of these bursae is complex and somewhat controversial.

The gluteus minimus bursa lies above and slightly anterior to the proximal superior surface of the greater trochanter. Two bursae are also identified deep to the gluteus minimus tendon: the primary and secondary subgluteus minimus bursae. The primary subgluteus minimus bursa is located deep to the anterior border of the gluteus minimus tendon as it inserted onto the anterior aspect of the GT, near its apex. The secondary subgluteus minimus bursa is usually found deep to the tendinous insertion of the gluteus minimus onto the anterolateral aspect of the GT.

The subgluteus medius bursa lies beneath the gluteus medius muscle, situated posterior and superior to the proximal edge of the greater trochanter.

The subgluteus maximus bursa lies beneath the converging fibers to the tensor fasciae latae and the gluteus maximus muscle and fascia as they join to form the iliotibial tract, and it separates the converging fibers from the greater trochanter and the origin of the vastus lateralis. It is lateral to the greater trochanter and is separated from the trochanter by the gluteus medius muscle.

Although variable, the subgluteus maximus is typically subdivided into up to 4 separate bursas. The deep subgluteus maximus bursa is the largest and most consistent of these subdivisions, often referred to as the "trochanteric bursa" and is often implicated in cases of symptomatic bursitis [10]. Other reported components of the subgluteus maximus bursas include the secondary deep, superficial, and gluteofemoral bursas.

The secondary deep subgluteus maximus bursa is often present in the same plane as the dominant deep subgluteus maximus bursa, posterior to the dominant deep bursa. The superficial subgluteus maximus bursa is positioned superficial to the deep bursa and is attached to overlying tissues.

The gluteofemoral bursa is positioned caudal to the GT and deep and superficial subgluteus bursae, and adhered to the iliotibial band (ITB) in the area where the tendinous fibers of the gluteus maximus inserted.

Deep to the gluteus medius tendon, on the anterior surface of the GT, three bursae are located. The two major bursae were the anterior subgluteus medius bursa and the piriformis bursa. A secondary piriformis bursa is often found. The anterior subgluteus medius bursa is generally located deep to the gluteus medius tendon, and anterior to the piriformis bursa and apex of the GT.

The piriformis bursa (also know as posterior subgluteus medius bursa) tended to be found at the insertion of the piriformis muscle at the apex of the GT.

The greater trochanter arises from the junction of the femoral neck and shaft. It is the site of attachment for 5 muscles, the gluteus medius and gluteus minimus tendons laterally and the piriformis, obturator externus and obturator internus more medially. As recently noted by Robertson et al., [21] the gluteus medius tendon has 2 distinct and consistent insertion sites on the greater trochanter, one on the lateral facet and the other on the superoposterior facet. The tendinous portion inserted on the superoposterior facet was noted to be stout with a circular shape, while that inserted on the lateral facet was larger and rectangular in shape.

Anterior to the gluteus medius insertion lies the insertion of the capsular and long heads of the gluteus minimus tendon on the anterior facet of the greater trochanter [22]. Superficial to the gluteus medius and minimus tendons lies a fibromuscular sheath composed of the gluteus maximus, tensor fascia lata, and ITB.

The iliotibial tract inserts in the iliac crest, overlies the greater trochanter, inserts indirectly in the lateral femoral condyle and reaches its distal insertion in the lateral tuberosity of the tibia (Gerdy's tubercle). Tensor fascia lata arises in the vicinity of the anterior superior iliac spine and inserts in, or descends as an anterior fascicle of, the iliotibial tract [23].

Gluteus maximus, the hallmark of bipedality, has an extensive origin in the iliac bone behind the posterior gluteal line, the sacrotuberous ligament, the thoracolumbar fascia, the sacrum and the coccix [24,25]. The superficial fibers and the upper deep part of this muscle merge into the iliotibial tract while its lower deep fibers insert in the gluteal tuberosity of the femur. Thus, two muscles attach in the iliotibial tract, one anteriorly and the other posteriorly, at or just distal to the greater trochanter.

The next layer is comprised of two overlapping muscles, gluteus medius and gluteus minimus. Gluteus medius has a wide origin on the surface of the iliac bone between the anterior and the posterior gluteal lines and inserts in 3 facets in the greater trochanter, the anterior, the lateral and the posterosuperior [26].

Gluteus minimus, which is covered by the former, also arises from the iliac bone below the anterior gluteal line and inserts in the anterior facet of the greater trochanter and partially in the joint capsule. Gluteus medius, gluteus minimus and tensor fascia lata stabilize the pelvis, and abduct and internally rotate the hip. Gluteus maximus also stabilizes the pelvis, helps in abducting the hip, and is an external rotator and an extensor of the hip. Tensor fascia lata, gluteus medius and gluteus minimus are innervated by the superior gluteal nerve that exits the pelvis above piriformis and runs between the latter two muscles. This nerve, particularly the branch for tensor fascia lata, runs quite close to the greater trochanter and may be damaged during surgical procedures [27].

Gluteus maximus is innervated by the inferior gluteal nerve which exits the pelvis below piriformis. The greater trochanter receives sensory innervation by a branch of the femoral nerve that approaches the trochanter from its back [28].

The ischial tuberosity is the site of origin of the long head of biceps femoris, semitendinosus and semimembranous. This can be attested by palpation of one's ischion while standing and flexing the knee. The long head of biceps and semitendinosus insert in the posteromedial surface of the ischial tuberosity and semimembranosus in its anterolateral surface [29]. These muscles extend the hip and because their insertion is below the knee they are also knee flexors. The ischions are covered by the glutei maximi in the standing position but in the sitting position these muscles move to the sides leaving the ischial tuberosities unprotected. Thus, weight is discharged on the ischion and the surrounding tissues. Excessive load at this site may lead to the formation of an adventitious bursa, the ischiogluteal bursa [30]. The increased popularity of hip endoscopy has improved the understanding of the anatomy of the peritrochanteric space [1,31]. The borders of the endoscopic lateral, peripheral, or peritrochanteric compartment consist of the tensor fascia lata and ITB laterally, the abductor tendons superomedially, the vastus lateralis inferomedially, the gluteus maximus muscle superiorly and its tendon posteriorly. Typically, the peripheral compartment is viewed with the operative leg off traction through the anterior portal, which is created 1-cm lateral to the anterior superior iliac spine in the interval between the sartorius and the tensor fascia lata [1,31]. The cannula is directed toward the greater trochanter with the leg in full extension, neutral adduction/abduction and 10 to 15 degree of internal rotation. The initial endoscopic view includes the insertion of the gluteus maximus into the posterior border of the ITB, the longitudinal fibers of the vastus lateralis and bursal tissue overlying the greater trochanter. In cases of severe trochanteric bursitis, this tissue may be hypertrophied, thick, and very vascular. Subsequent to the clearing of the bursal tissue with a motorized shaver and/or radiofrequency probe (through a distal posterior portal placed halfway between the tip of the greater trochanter and the vastus tubercle along the posterior one-third of the greater trochanteric midline), continued inspection will identify the fibers of the gluteus medius as it inserts onto the greater trochanter. This insertion is carefully examined for evidence of full or partial-thickness tears. Finally, the ITB is assessed, particularly the posterior one-third, looking for evidence of abrasive wear consistent with external coxa saltans.

Physiopathology

The causes of GTPS can be traumatic and nontraumatic. Risk factors are various and variously described, including age older than 40 years, female gender, ipsilateral ITB pain, knee osteoarthritis (OA), obesity, and low back pain (LBP) [17,32].

In an observational study, Schapira et al., [17] found that 91.6% of patients diagnosed with trochanteric bursitis had other associated pathological conditions, such as peripheral OA, rheumatoid arthritis, meralgia paresthetica and lumbosacral OA. The increased prevalence in women may be attributed to altered biomechanics associated with differences in the size, shape, and orientation of the pelvis (gynecoid vs android), and its association with relative knee valgus and hip varus. This may result in higher tensile stresses to the iliotibial tract and hip abductors, predisposing them to injury.

Obesity may be a contributing risk factor by the combined effect of increased stress on the hip joint, hip and knee OA and low back pain [9]. Because trochanteric bursitis (TB) can result from friction between the bursae and GT, it frequently occurs with overuse, microtrauma or regional muscle dysfunction [33,34]. However, misdiagnosis is common.

Specific etiologies of GTPS include repetitive activity, acute trauma, crystal deposition and infection, especially tuberculosis [9,35,36]. Finally, intrinsic degenerative tendinosis (also called angiofibroblastic tendinosis) also occurs in the hip abductors. Calcifications about the greater trochanter have been reported in 13% to 40% of patients with chronic GTPS [7,17]. A number of authors have found that peritrochanteric calcifications are typically located at the gluteus tendon insertions rather than in the bursae [7,17]. The presence of calcific tendinoses in the hip abductors suggests that intrinsic degenerative tendinopathy occurs in chronic GTPS.

When an inciting event can be identified, the initial pathology usually occurs at tendinous attachments to the GT, with secondary involvement of adjacent bursae [13]. In cases of acute trauma or the presence of other risk factors, extra caution should be exercised so that a more serious condition, such as femoral neck stress fracture or avascular necrosis is not misdiagnosed as TB [34,37]. Such repetitive, cumulative irritation often occurs in runners but can also be seen in less active individuals. Other predisposing factors include a leg-length discrepancy (dynamic evaluations for limb length inequalities are likely to be more important than static observations on the examination) and lateral hip surgery [34,38].

The main tendon of the gluteus medius muscle attaches to the postero-superior aspect of the GT, with the lateral tendon inserting into the lateral aspect. The gluteus minimus muscle attaches to the anterior facet of the GT. Consequently, inflammation and tears of either the gluteus medius or minimus muscles, or their tendinous insertions, from tension imposed by the ITB and/or frictional trauma from overuse, may result in GTPS [39].

Bunker et al., [40] reported that gluteus medius and minimus tears occurred most commonly in the anterior aspect near their insertions on the greater trochanter and were usually interstitial or deeper-surfaced tears having a circular or oval appearance with rolled, mature edges. The underlying bone showed reactive sclerotic changes, osteophytes, and cysts [40].

In 2008, Silva et al., [38] reported on pathologic specimens from patients diagnosed with "trochanteric bursitis" after trochanteric bursectomy. Their bursal specimens revealed fibroadipose tissue with no signs of acute or chronic inflammation.

These findings strongly suggest that, at least in long-standing GTPS, bursal inflammation does not play a causative role in pain. Additionally the tendinosis encountered in GTPS is likely due to a process intrinsic to the tendon itself.

In the study by Bunker et al., [40], gluteus medius tears were reported to be interstitial or deep surface tears. If the primary pathology was external impingement against the iliotibial tract, the tendon lesions would be expected to be on the superficial surface instead.

In chronic cases of GTPS, the initial pathology is often gluteal tendinopathy, with trochanteric bursitis more likely being secondary and reactive [41]. External impingement may occur, but this is often a secondary effect of myotendinous dysfunction and resulting mechanical derangements.

Clinical Evaluation

GTPS is characterized by chronic, intermittent aching pain at the greater trochanteric region at the lateral hip and/or buttock that is exacerbated by lying on the affected side, with prolonged standing or transitioning to a standing position, sitting with the affected leg crossed and with climbing stairs, running or other high impact activities [42]. Any movement of the affected hip can reproduce the pain of greater trochanteric bursitis, but external rotation and abduction of the hip are most common. Approximately, 50% of patients experience pain radiating along the lateral aspect of the thigh to the knee, and occasionally below the knee [13]. Occasionally, patients experience numbness in the upper thigh with no specific dermatomal pattern. Invariably, there is tenderness along the lateral or posterior aspect of the GT [33,38].

Pain extending to the groin or down the lateral thigh that mimics lumbar disk herniation ((i.e., pseudoradiculopathy) may be reported by some individuals [8,32,43].

Pain radiation patterns may complicate the diagnosis of GTPS because of anatomical overlap with the iliotibial tract and mid-lumbar dermatomes (L2–4) [8]. Not only nerve roots, but radiation patterns from other structures in the lumbar spine, sacroiliac joint, and intervertebral discs and ligaments, can replicate TB [44-46]. In addition, damage to the nerve supply of surrounding structures may elicit neuropathic symptoms that can simulate GTPS. These nerve structures include the inferior gluteal nerve, which innervates the gluteus maximus muscles and is formed from the ventral rami of spinal nerves L5–S2, and the superior gluteal nerve, which derives from the L4–S1 nerve roots and innervates the superior aspect of the femoral neck, tensor fascia lata, and the gluteus medius and minimus muscles [19].

The most common disability is exercise limitations to include walking. It is also associated with broken sleep patterns secondary to the inability to lie on the affected side because of pain. In addition, a large number of patients have bilateral bursitis, further sleep interrupting patterns.

The physical examination of a patient with GTPS characteristically reveals point tenderness in the posterolateral area of the GT [8]. Typically, this will be at either the site of the gluteus medius tendon insertion [13,15,33] or in a more cephalad position overlying the insertion of the gluteus minimus tendon on a ridge lateral to the anterior triangular area of the GT [13,22]. While the patient is standing, palpate the lateral hip area in a cephalic direction beginning below the greater trochanter eminence until the area of maximal tenderness is identified ("jump sign") [47].

Passive hip flexion with abduction, external rotation, and extension (the so-called Patrick or FABERE test) may reproduce symptoms. To perform resisted abduction, place the patient in a sitting position with knees flexed. The examiner places his or her hand on the lateral aspect of the upper thigh and instructs the patient to move the thigh laterally against the resistance. External rotation of the hip is obtained by placing the patient in a sitting position with the knees flexed and adducting the lower leg (shin). If there was direct trauma to the area, abrasions or ecchymoses may be evident.

Krout and Anderson have proposed a set of diagnostic criteria that were later modified by Rasmussen and Fano [48]. In these criteria, the first 2 plus 1 of the remaining criteria have to be present to diagnose trochanteric bursitis: 1) lateral hip pain; 2) tenderness about the greater trochanter; 3) pain at the extremes of rotation, abduction, or adduction, especially a positive Patrick-fabere test; 4) pain on strong contraction of hip abductors; and 5) pseudoradiculopathy, mainly pain radiating down the lateral aspect of the thigh. Although these criteria are sound and appear consistent with clinical practice, their sensitivity, specificity, and predictive value have not been established [4].

Pain on flexion and extension of the hip is indicative of intra-articular hip disease and not usually of a greater trochanteric bursitis [49]. Objective swelling is rare because of the bulky muscles overlying the deep structures of the trochanter bursa.

Causes of lateral hip pain, such as ITB syndrome and meralgia paresthetica, are common regional pain syndromes that can be differentiated from GTPS by physical examination signs, such as a positive Ober's test and sensory deficits, respectively.

Lateral hip pain produced with active internal rotation, active external rotation, or resisted abduction, at 45° of hip flexion, suggests gluteus medius or gluteus minimus dysfunction. A positive 30-s single-leg stance test, in which pain was reproduced while standing on the affected limb for 30 s, was 100% sensitive and 97.3% specific for gluteal tendinopathy [50]. The resisted external derotation test, in which the 90- flexed hip and knee is held with the hip in external rotation and then resisted as the patient attempts to return the limb to neutral rotation, was 88% sensitive and 97.3% specific for gluteal tendinopathy when lateral hip pain was reproduced [50]. In most patients with limitation of range of motion of the affected hip, the underlying cause is arthritis. Other physical findings such as limited lumbar range of motion and muscle atrophy may reveal other associated conditions such as lumbar spondylosis and nerve root compression. In severe cases of bursitis the presence of soft tissue crepitus can be found [51].

Additionally a positive Trendelenburg test, abnormal lateral pelvic tilt while assuming a single-legged stance on the symptomatic limb, can aid in detecting gluteus medius tears, with 73% sensitivity and 77% specificity [52]. In Bird et al., [52] only Trendelenburg's sign (kappa 0.67) and pain on resisted hip abduction (kappa 0.62) had good interobserver agreement.

Imaging

The investigation of hip bursitis is poorly described in the literature, with a number of case study articles [53-55] predominating. This is, at least in part, because of the poor understanding of the pathology behind the syndrome. As the understanding of the heterogeneous nature of the underlying cause of GTPS has improved, a number of studies have been conducted to assess the efficacy of ultrasonography (US) [56], magnetic resonance imaging (MRI) [41,50,52,57-60], bone scintigraphy [61] and plain radiography [62] in identifying different pathologies.

No specific radiographic findings are of diagnostic value for a trochanteric bursitis [63]. X-Rays of the hip, pelvis, and lower spine may show evidence of one or more of the associated musculoskeletal conditions. Plain x-rays are often negative.

On occasion (figure 1), calcifications around the greater trochanter may be seen (approximately 40% of patients with greater trochanteric bursitis) [64]. These calcifications varies in size and shape from a few millimeters to 3 to 4 cm in diameter. They appear as linear or small, rounded masses that are separated or grouped together. Irregularities can also be seen on the surface of the greater trochanter. Plain film radiography may show radio-opacities suggesting calcific tendinopathy or bursopathy. Trochanteric exostoses or osteophytes may be seen in long-standing cases of GTPS. Radiographs are often useful in assessing for osteoarthrosis, FAI, or bony avulsions as well. .

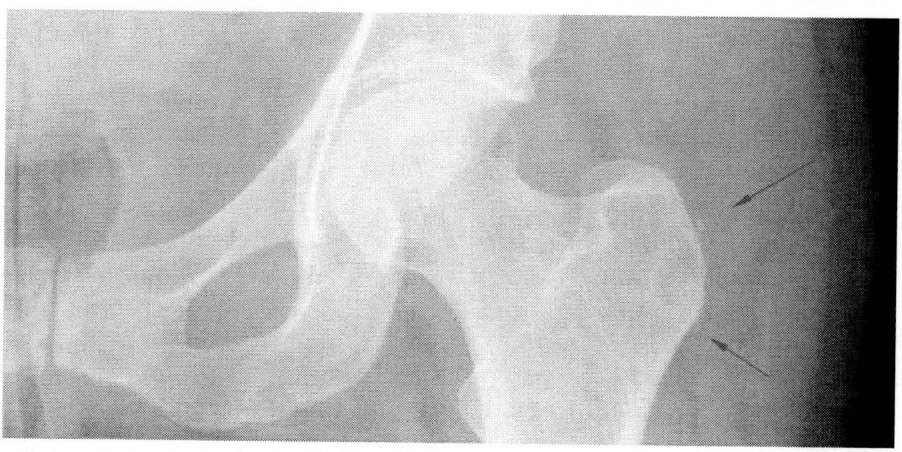

Figure 1. medius gluteus and vastus lateralis ossifications.

Steinert et al., [62] assessed the correlation between MRI and plain radiograph findings of the hip in patients with abductor tendon abnormalities. They concluded that pronounced (>2 mm) surface irregularities of the greater trochanter on conventional radiographs are associated with abductor tendon MR abnormalities and peri-tendinous oedema.

Musculoskeletal US is emerging as an accurate, cost-effective, readily available, and easily applied imaging modality in musculoskeletal medicine. Its most significant limitation, however, is that its diagnostic value is very operator dependent. In a recent study, Fearon et al., [56] showed that, in skilled hands, ultrasonography had a high positive predictive value for peritrochanteric abnormalities. Degenerative changes to the gluteus tendons can be visualized as tenohypertrophy, heteroechogenicity, neovascularity, and disturbed tendon architecture on ultrasonography. Partial-thickness and full-thickness tendon tears are seen directly as hypoechoic or anechoic foci or indirectly as contour defects, through transmission enhancement, or edge artifacts. Bursal effusions are seen as large anechoic collections.

For tendinopathies, the concept of the four greater trochanter facets is well demonstrated by US aiding in correct identification of the affected tendons [19,39]. The gluteus minimus and gluteus medius tendons attach onto the anterior and lateral facets, respectively. The gluteus minimus insertion is variable and ranges from a triangular to an irregular L shape at the anterior facet.

Most patients exhibit abnormalities in the anterior and posterior portion of the gluteus medius; an effusion inside the trochanteric bursa can be an associated finding. US signs of gluteal tendinopathy are based on the development of different tendinotic stages. Tendinosis is defined by a loss of fibrillar echotexture, loss of echogenicity due to edema and mucoid degeneration, heterogeneous echogenicity, altogether often present with tendon thickening that can be diffuse or focal. The tendon of the gluteus minimus or the anterior and posterior tendons of the gluteus medius can be involved alone or in association. However, the anterior portion of the gluteus medius is the most commonly affected; only a minority of patients show changes in the gluteus minimus [65]. Increased vascularity on color Doppler is an uncommon finding [66]. The affected tendon may be tender to sonopalpation. Calcific tendinosis within the gluteal tendons or at the insertion in terms of enthesopathy can be further present and is better seen on US than MRI by showing hyperechoic welldefined or ill-defined echogenic depositions. US can be used to guide aspiration to treat these calcifications.

Coxa saltans is described as an audible and potentially painful snapping of the hip during activities that require repetitive flexion, extension, and abduction [67-69]. The external variety of snapping hip syndrome involves the soft tissues overlying the greater trochanter, most typically the ITB but also the anterior border of the gluteus maximus. When the hip is in a position of extension, the ITB lies posterior to the greater trochanter. Snapping of the IT band can occur during hip flexion activities when the IT band glides over the greater trochanter to lie in an anterior position. Although gliding of the IT band over the greater trochanter is physiologic and a benign, asymptomatic snapping hip can be present especially in athletes, occasionally the snapping leads to inflammation and pain, significantly limiting affected patients activities [68,69]. Patients with symptomatic external snapping hip tend to be in their late teenage years or early twenties and frequently report active lifestyles.

A diagnosis of symptomatic external coxa saltans is typically evident based on the patient's presenting history. The typical case presents with a painful, snapping sensation localizing to the region about the greater trochanter.

Although a history of a traumatic event precipitating the snapping may be present, this is less common than an atraumatic insidious symptom onset. Physical examination of suspected cases of external snapping hip usually starts with placing the patient on their side with the affected leg up [68]. The patient is then asked to actively flex their hip whereas the examiner palpates the greater trochanter feeling the snapping of the IT band. The diagnosis can be confirmed if pressure applied over the proximal aspect of the greater trochanter prevents snapping with repeated hip flexion. Diagnostic imaging usually begins with plain radiographs of the affected hip looking for evidence of loose bodies or synovial chondromatosis, which can be causes of the internal variety of coxa saltans. However, similar to cases of trochanteric bursitis or abductor tendon pathology, plain x-rays are typically negative. Real-time dynamic ultrasound can be used to visualize the snapping phenomenon and associated bursitis whereas at the same time ruling out other sources of pain [43].

Tendon tears are manifested by tendon thinning and partial or full-thickness anechoic defects within the tendon. Partial-thickness tears typically involve the deep portion of the anterior gluteus medius tendon [65]. Ruptures can also be found at the insertion and in the tendon substance itself. In full-thickness tears, the tendon appears retracted proximally with anechoic effusion related to the hematoma seen between it and the naked greater trochanter filling the trochanteric bursa. A "bold" facet with absence of tendon fibers is compatible with a complete tear. Musclewasting may also be evident with loss of muscle bulk and increased echogenicity due to fat replacement. In the presence of cortical irregularities deep to the gluteal insertions, a careful evaluation of the overlying tendon, should be performed to visualize a potential partial-thickness tear.

Ultrasound can also be used to evaluate the abductor tendons, identifying thickening and fluid consistent with tendinosis or the presence of partial or full thickness tears [65,66].

In bursitis, acute bursal fluid collections are readily appreciated as a hypoechoic thin fluid accumulation. Fluid distension of the trochanteric bursa appears as a well-circumscribed crescent shaped hypoechoic to anechoic collection located at the lateral aspect of the greater trochanter deep to the gluteus maximus, which can extend superficially over the posterior insertion of the gluteus medius. Chronic bursitis, which is commonly present in chronic tendon disease, can show effusions as well; however, isoechoic bursal wall thickening can be present that might be easily overlooked. Symptoms in these conditions might be prevalent due to adhesions of the bursal layers. It is not always possible to differentiate trochanteric bursitis from an underlying tendinopathy, and, in many instances, the two conditions can coexist.

Trochanteric bursitis can be interpreted as a true impingement syndrome [70] from the pathophysiologic point of view. In addition, in hip abductor tendons tear, impingement of the greater trochanter on the fasciae latae may develop, thus sustaining chronic bursitis. Again, especially in these cases, sonopalpation is of great diagnostic value.

Fearon et al., [56] compared US results to intraoperative findings in 24 patients. US had a sensitivity of 0.79 and positive predictive value of 1.0 of diagnosing a tear in either the gluteus medius or minimus tendon. Based on the postoperative histological findings, US had a sensitivity of 0.61, a specificity of 1.0, a positive predictive value of 1.0 and a negative predictive value of 1.0 of diagnosing bursa pathology. They suggested that these results confirm US as a clinically useful tool in GTPS, with intraoperative findings that show tendinopathy and bursal pathology to co-exist in GTPS.

MRI provides high-resolution imaging of the complex peritrochanteric anatomy (figures 2-3). MRI may show degenerative changes to the gluteus medius and gluteus minimus tendons as abnormal T2 signal change with disturbed tendon architecture on T1-weighted imaging [57]. Tears of the gluteus medius can be interstitial, partial thickness or full thickness, with full-thickness tears tending to be large in size [21,66].

Partial-thickness and fullthickness tears in the hip abductors - and in the older population, muscle atrophy, and fatty degeneration - can easily be seen on MRI [47]. T2 signal change consistent with trochanteric bursopathy may be evident, but this is not usually seen in isolation.

The MRI appearance of tendinosis and tear of the abductor tendons of the hip is the same as in other locations and includes alterations in tendon signal and caliber [66].

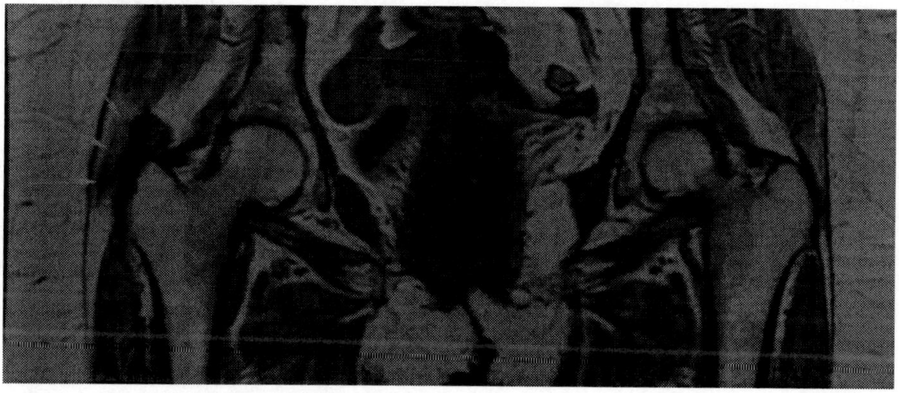

Figure 2. trochanteric bursitis (MRI view).

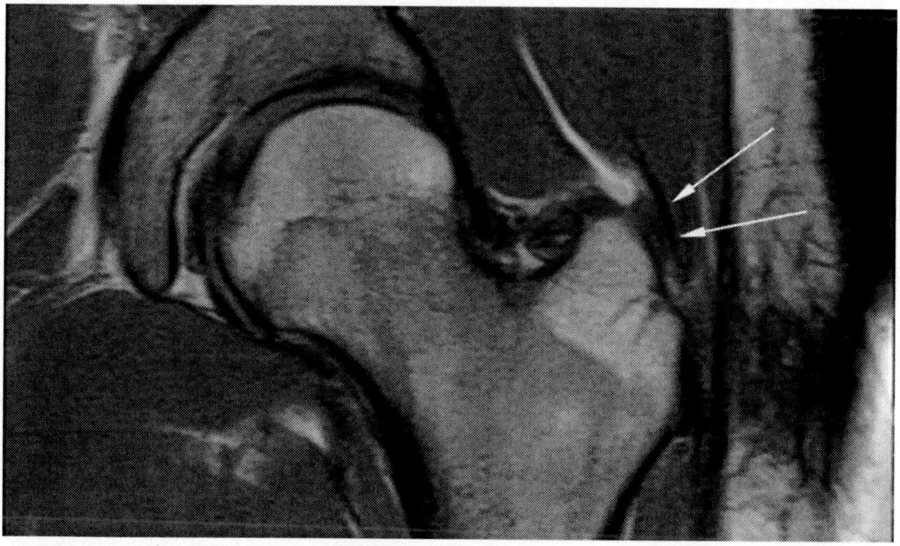

Figure 3. medius gluteus tendinopaty (MRI view).

Muscle atrophy is frequent with chronic large tears [59]. If a larger field of view is utilized to incorporate both hips, tendon visualization is often limited and secondary signs become critical in detecting abductor tendon tears. The most frequently encountered secondary sign is a greater than 1 cm in diameter localized area of high signal superior to the greater trochanter [59,66].

In a retrospective evaluation of 74 hip MRIs comparing findings from 15 surgically proven cases of abductor tears and 59 controls, Cvitanic et al., [58] have shown a 91% accuracy in the MRI diagnosis of gluteus medius and minimus tears. In this review, consistent signs of abductor tears were MRI evidence of increased T2 signal superior and lateral to the greater trochanter and evidence of tendon discontinuity on T1 images.

Bird et al., [52] and Woodley et al., [60] compared MRI results with specific clinical tests. Both studies looked at the specificity and sensitivity of a positive Trendelenberg's test in predicting gluteal tendon pathology. Bird et al., [52] recorded a specificity of 76.9% and sensitivity of 72.7% in their trial of 24 cases, Woodley et al., [60] achieved a specificity of 94%, but a sensitivity of only 23%, in 40 patients. Bird et al., [52] also looked at pain on resisted hip abduction (sensitivity of 72.7%, specificity of 46.2%) and pain on resisted hip internal rotation (sensitivity of 54.5% and specificity of 69.2%). Woodley et al., [60] found that the highest specificity and sensitivity was provided by decreased gluteus medius and minimus strength (sensitivity 80%, specificity 71%). Bone scintigraphy is another imaging modality. In a prognostic study, Walker et al., [61] assessed scintigraphic criteria for the diagnosis of trochanteric bursitis and evaluated the relationship of trochanteric bursitis to gluteus medius tendonitis and lumbar degenerative disease in predicting symptom relapse after corticosteroid injection.

Scintigraphic criteria had a positive predictive value of 90% and a negative predictive value of 97% for the diagnosis of trochanteric bursitis and gluteus medius tendon disease.

Although no data meta-analysis can be performed, qualitatively, MRI appears to be the most effective method of imaging hip bursitis. There is a consistently strong correlation between intraoperative findings and imaging interpretation. Allied to this are the encouraging results of the individual studies assessing US and plain radiography, which may be useful adjuncts to MRI.

Conservative Treatment

Initially, treatment of greater trochanteric bursitis, coxa saltans or tendon tears involves ice, nonsteroidal anti-inflammatory drugs (NSAIDs) to reduce pain and inflammation, weight loss ,and activity modification (e.g., avoiding stairs, reducing repetitive sit-to-stand movements) [45]. The use of nonsteroidal inflammatory drugs (NSAIDs) is controversial in GTPS. While effective as analgesics, long-term NSAID use has been shown to hamper tendon healing elsewhere in the body (e.g., shoulder) [71]. Given the central role of gluteus dysfunction and tendinosis in GTPS, the potential detrimental effects of NSAIDs should not be overlooked. NSAIDs may be beneficial in acute cases but should be avoided in chronic cases of gluteal tendinopathy.

The individual is instructed to avoid placing direct pressure on the bursa by sleeping on the unaffected side and using a pillow between the knees (adductor pillow) to minimize indirect bursal compression from overlying tight musculature.

Physical therapy focusing on stretching, flexibility, strengthening, and gait mechanics [10,17,43], is also usefull. Soft tissue mobilization and massage may be helpful for gluteal trigger points. In the rehabilitation of GTPS, stretching and maintaining normal hip range-of-motion are important; these include both passive and active stretching, including neuromuscular facilitation techniques. Iliotibial tract and tensor fascia lata contractures should be addressed with stretching as well. Painful eccentric strengthening (strengthening a muscle-tendon unit while lengthening the unit) has been shown to improve outcomes in degenerative tendinoses in other areas of the body, including hamstring, rotator cuff, elbow, patellar, and Achilles tendons [72-75]. It is likely that similar improvements in pain, function, and activity tolerance could be attained with eccentric rehabilitation of gluteal tendinosis. Given the importance of the hip abductors in core stabilization, a focus on flexibility, strength, and endurance of the other core and pelvic stabilizing muscles is appropriate. It is also reasonable to address potential biomechanical contributors to GTPS. Pes planus and foot overpronation could be addressed with taping, strapping, or orthoses. Individuals with iliotibial tract contractures and engaged in running or other repetitive activities may find some relief with counterforce bracing, taping, or strapping.

If the individual has developed an altered gait pattern to reduce pain (antalgic gait pattern), gait training may be necessary to restore normal movement patterns with ambulation. In severe cases, temporary use of an assistive device (cane, crutch) may be necessary.

When these interventions fail, bursa or lateral hip injections performed with corticosteroid and local anesthetics (24 mg betamethasone and 1% lidocaine, or equivalent) have been shown to provide pain relief, with response rates ranging from 60% to 100% [12,13,48,76-78]. Although there are no placebo-controlled trials evaluating the efficacy of corticosteroid injection therapy, several prospective studies have been published [77].

In a study of 75 patients with trochanteric bursitis treated with lidocaine/bethamethasone injections, Shbeeb et al., [77] reported that 77.1% had pain relief at 1 week of follow-up with 61.3% of patients continuing to be symptom free at 6 months. For patients who respond to an initial injection but have later return of their symptoms, a repeat injection into the peritrochanteric space may be used successfully [10].

Rasmussen and Fano [48] evaluated 36 patients after corticosteroid injections for simple trochanteric bursitis. Twenty-four patients reported excellent results after one or two local corticosteroid injections, improvement was observed in the remaining cases but nine patients relapsed within 2 years.

Karpinsky et al., [79] reviewed 15 patients undergoing local steroid injection for pain and tenderness at the tip of the greater trochanter. Twelve patients reported great improvement once injected. Of the three patients complaining of little or no relief, two responded to ultrasound and massage. Improvement was usually permanent and there were no relapses.

In a multicentre double-blind randomized controlled trial, Cohen et al., [80] assessed outcomes of two groups of patients who received corticosteroid injections with (fluoroscopy group) and without (blind group) fluoroscopic guidance. No significant inter-group difference was noted. One month after injection the average pain scores were 2.7 at rest and 5.0 with activity in the fluoroscopy group compared with 2.2 and 4.0 in the blind injection group. Three months after the injection, 15 (47%) patients in the blind group and 13 (41%) in the fluoroscopy group continued to have a positive outcome.

Transcutaneous electrical neuromuscular stimulation (TENS), ionophoresis and therapeutic ultrasound may be helpful in some cases for pain relief [81]. The physical therapist focuses on stretching exercises to improve hip range of motion, especially external rotation, and to increase the extensibility of adjacent tight soft tissues (e.g., gluteus medius, iliotibial band, tensor fascia lata) that may be causing friction on the inflamed bursa.

The addition of low-energy ESWT (external shpck wave therapy) has been shown to improve both pain and hip function in patients with GTPS failing an initial trial of nonoperative conservative treatment. These benefits were demonstrated by Furia et al., [82] in a group of patients with GTPS at 1, 3, and 12 months. Rompe et al., [83] have shown benefit up to 15 months. Presumably, ESWT works on the basis of stimulating a healing inflammatory response in degenerative tendinosis. When ESWT was compared with a home training regimen, there was moderate evidence that it was as effective at 1 and

15 months in relieving pain and improving function, but effectiveness was better at 4 months [83]. Rompe et al., [83] provided moderate evidence that ESWT was less effective than corticosteroid injections at 1 month, but with time, it became more effective at 4 and 15 months after intervention. Moreover, ESWT had a 74% success rate at 15 months compared with 35% for the injection. These results indicate that ESWT is a viable short- and long-term treatment option for GTPS.

Considered alternatives to more costly surgical procedures, other interventions for chronic degenerative tendinosis include regenerative and proliferative injection therapies. While studies on the effectiveness of these procedures have lacked consistency, their use in treating various tendinopathies is growing in popularity (including the Achilles tendon, patellar tendon, and lateral epicondyle of the elbow [84-89]. To date, the use of these therapies in the treatment of GTPS, specifically, has not been well studied. As in ESWT, the aim of these treatments is to rekindle the healing inflammatory response, promote the influx of peripheral stem cells and reparative mediators, and encourage the collagen regenerative and remodeling processes. Prolotherapy involves the injection of nonorganic substances to elicit this response. Regenerative injection therapy involves the injection of biologic, usually autologous, tissue grafts. Examples include autologous whole blood, platelet-rich plasma concentrates, processed lipoaspirate concentrates, and bone marrow aspirate concentrates. While these procedures can be done via surface anatomy landmarks, ultrasonographic needle guidance helps to ensure precision and higher effectiveness [90]. Given the inconsistency in reported efficacy, more research on regenerative and proliferative therapies is needed.

Surgical Treatment

In patients who fail conservative treatment, surgical intervention has been advocated: open bursectomy with an unsutured iliotibial band incision [91], excision of a portion of the iliotibial band overlying the greater trochanter and removal of the bursa [92], debridement and repair of damaged gluteal tendons with resection of the bursa [50,93], iliotibial band Z-lengthening and removal of the bursa with tendon repair [94], endoscopic bursectomy [95], endoscopic bursectomy with debridement of damaged gluteal tendons [96], and endoscopic bursectomy with concomitant iliotibial band release [95].

In endoscopic view several portals have been described, but the anterior portal seems to be the best portal to access the peritrochanteric space and is created 1-cm lateral to the anterior superior iliac spine and in the interval between tensor fascia lata and sartorius. The leg is placed in complete extension and roughly 15 degree of abduction. A 5.0-mm metallic cannula is positioned between the ITB and the lateral aspect of the greater trochanter, and the tip of the cannula can be used to sweep proximal and distal to ensure placement in the proper location. Fluoroscopy can also be used to confirm that the cannula is located immediately adjacent to the greater trochanter. The 30-degree arthroscope can be introduced into the cannula and the lens is directed to view distally.

The initial view should visualize the insertion of the gluteus maximus into the posterior border the ITB. The distal peritrochanteric space portal (DPSP) can be established under needle localization and approximately midway between the tip of the greater trochanter and vastus tubercle along the posterior one-third of the greater trochanter midline. A mechanical shaver can be placed into the peritrochanteric space through the DPSP to begin the bursectomy, and radiofrequency energy device can be used intermittently for hemostasis. The gluteus minimus tendon and muscle is visualized anteriorly with the arthroscope and light source directed anterosuperior. When the arthroscope is directed superiorly, the gluteus medius tendon insertion into the greater trochanter can be visualized lying posterior to the gluteus minimus. Any overlying bursa should be debrided, which will also facilitate exposure of the gluteus medius and minimus insertions. The arthroscope should also be directed toward the ITB, and the posterior one-third ITB can be evaluated for evidence of snapping ITB or abrasive wear or erythema to the tendons overlying the greater trochanter.

Trochanteric Bursitis

Several types of surgical procedures are available to treat trochanteric bursitis [10]. The primary goal of all procedures designed to treat this condition is to remove the thickened bursa, to remove any bone spurs that may have formed on the greater trochanter, and to relax the large tendon of the gluteus maximus. Surgical options include open or endoscopic bursectomy and ITB release.

Endoscopic bursectomy [81,95-98] may be performed in either the lateral decubitus or supine positions [3]. In the lateral position, bursectomy can be performed through a proximal portal 2-cm posterior to the tip of the trochanter and a distal portal at the postero-inferior margin of the bursa.

Debridement can be performed with a 4-mm full-radius resector placed in the proximal portal. When the bursectomy is complete, the arthroscope and shaver are switched for a final check. If there is an associated prominence of the greater trochanter, the bone can be shaved with a 5.5-mm burr.

The open surgical procedure consisted of simple longitudinal release of the iliotibial band over the greater trochanter and excision of the subgluteal bursa: an incision approximately 10 cm long centred over the greater trochanter is made in line with the femoral shaft. An area of the iliotibial band 4–5 cm wide by approximately 15 cm long overlying the greater trochanter is exposed. Longitudinal incisions are made anteriorly and posteriorly and the band divided in a Z-fashion. The flaps are reflected and the bursa identified and resected.

A tear in the tendon of gluteus medius is easily seen, with a bald area seen on the anterior part of the greater trochanter. However, tears in gluteus minimus are difficult to see without splitting the gluteus medius. The longitudinal incision in the iliotibial band is then repaired by lengthening the band by approximately 1 cm. Proximally, a 5-cm defect is left open overlying the posterior aspect of the greater trochanter.

In a prospective study, Baker et al., [96] investigated the effectiveness of endoscopic trochanteric bursectomy for recalcitrant TB in 30 patients. The mean pain score improved from a visual analog scale score of 7.2 preoperatively to 3.1 at final follow-up (mean, 26.1 months). In another prospective study, Craig et al., [94] evaluated ITB lengthening for refractory TB in 15 patients (17 hips) with a mean follow-up of 47 months. Complete resolution of symptoms was reported in 8 of 17 patients, partial relief occurred in 8 patients, and 1 patient experienced no benefit.

Similar good results were reported by Fox et al., [81] in their retrospective review of 27 patients treated with endoscopic bursectomy. At a minimum of 1 year of follow-up, the investigators reported that 23 of the 27 patients had good or excellent results immediately after the procedure and had no postoperative complications. Symptom recurrence was reported in 2 patients (7.4%) at 5 years of clinical follow-up. Believing that the ITB is a major contributor to the pain, inflammation, and impingement leading to trochanteric bursitis, Farr et al., [95] describe including an IT band release with their endoscopic bursectomy. In 2 patients treated with this technique, the investigators report that both had complete symptom relief and returned to their occupational and recreational activities without recurrence.

In the study by Slawski and Howard [91], five active patients (7 hips) with refractory trochanteric bursitis received simple longitudinal release of the ITB (over the greater trochanter), and excision of the subgluteal bursa. Unresponsive to conservative measures as nonsteroidal anti-inflammatory medication, ITB stretching, diathermy, ultrasound and injections of local anesthetics combined with corticosteroids, all patients had experienced marked limitation in vocational and recreational activities. At an average post-operative assessment of 20 months, four of the 5 patients (six hips) had an average Harris Hip Score of 95.0, compared with an average baseline score of 51.7. All patients were satisfied with the surgical results and returned to unrestricted vocational and athletic activities. Concerning the remaining patients evaluated 6 months post-operatively, Harris Hip Score had improved from 49 to 84.

Dunbar et al., [99] reported that bursectomy and Z-lengthening has been shown to be an effective and long-term operative solution for the treatment of refractory trochanteric bursitis when conservative measures have failed.

Govaert et al., [100] purposed a trochanteric reduction osteotomy of 5–10 mm with distal and medial trochanteric fixation, as a treatment for refractory trochanteric bursitis. At a mean follow-up of 23.5 months, the mean Merle d'Aubigne´ and Postel score was improved from preoperative value of 15.8 to a post-operative score of 27.5. After surgery seven patients had no pain and two had mild pain during daily activities. The range of movement and the walking ability were normal in these patients and seven were satisfied with the results. The remaining three patients had tolerable pain with limited activity.

Septic bursitis is unusual in the hip bursa but does occur. The bursal fluid can be examined in the laboratory for the microorganisms causing the infection [101]. Septic bursitis is caused by the Staphylococcus aureus. This is confirmed by antibiogram from the fluid in the bursa and requires antibiotic treatment. When a patient has such a serious infection, there may be underlying causes. There could be undiscovered diabetes, or an inefficient immune system (e.g., human immunodeficiency virus infection, HIV) [102]. Repeated aspiration of the infected fluid may be required. Surgical drainage and removal of the infected bursa may also be necessary [94].

Tendon Tears

Although open techniques have been reported for gluteus medius and minimus tears noted during femoral neck fracture fixation and total hip arthroplasty, recent advances and experience with hip arthroscopy have led to endoscopic techniques for abductor tendon repair [1,21,103].

Two endoscopic repair techniques of the gluteus tendon have been described in the literature [3,18,103-106]. Voos et al., [103], described a technique to repair gluteus tendon tears via the peritrochanteric compartment utilizing an anterior portal and a distal posterior portal. Suture anchors can be placed into the footprint of the abductor tendons, the sutures are passed sequentially through the edges of the prepared gluteus medius tendon with a suture-passing device and tied.

In his case series study, Voos et al., [103] evaluated 10 patients after endoscopic repair of the gluteus medius tears. At an average follow-up of 25 months, all patients had no pain and had regained 5/5 motor strength in the hip abductors. Modified Harris Hip Scores at 1 year averaged 94 points (range, 84–100), and Hip Outcomes Scores averaged 93 points (range, 85–100). Seven of 10 patients said their hip was normal and 3 said their hip was nearly normal. [46]

Domb [106] described another endoscopic technique of approaching the tendon through a longitudinal split in line with its fibers, in order to visualize and treat intra-substance tears without affecting the integrity and strength of the tendon itself. He describes the use of posterolateral and distal peritrochanteric portals. This technique results in a side-to-side repair of the longitudinal tendon split while firmly approximating the tendon to the footprint on the lateral facet.

Open repair have also been described but to our knowledge there is only one study describing the results of this technique: Kagan et al., showed all patients were free of pain at a median follow up of 45 months (range, 21–60 months) [93].

Domb's procedure [106] appears more challenging for the surgeon and aims to better preserve the tendon, which may be helpful in younger and more active patients. Studies with a larger cohort are necessary to give an evidence-based conclusion for the efficacy of these repair techniques.

Coxa Saltans

For the rare patient with refractory snapping hip after an extensive attempt at nonoperative management, surgical intervention may be indicated.

Open iliotibial band release or lengthening has been the traditional surgical option to treat external snapping hip syndrome [67,69,100,107,108].

Ilizaliturri [109] has recently described a technique for endoscopic iliotibial band release performed under image intensifier control. He describes proximal and distal trochanteric portals through which either a Z- or a diamond-shaped release is performed. Where indicated, the additional treatment of gluteus medius tear, trochanteric bone prominence or bursitis may be performed as described subsequently. According to Ilizaliturri's review [110], endoscopic surgery in the peritrochanteric space seems safe, reproducible, and allows for the successful treatment of snapping hip syndromes.

Brignall and Stainsby reported good results in 8 patients treated with z-plasty, with all 8 having complete resolution of pain and snapping at a mean follow-up of 3 years [111]. In a review of 9 symptomatic snapping hips in 8 patients with a mean age of 25.6 years, Provencher et al., [69] described the results of IT band z-plasty. At a mean follow-up of 22.9 months the investigators reported that all 8 patients had complete resolution of their snapping hip symptoms, with 7 of the 8 returning to full, unrestricted activities. White et al., [67] described a new surgical approach for the treatment of refractory external coxa saltans, relaxing the resting tension in the IT band through transverse step cuts made along a 10-cm longitudinal incision placed in line with the fibers overlying the greater trochanter. In a review of 16 patients treated with this technique, the investigators reported that 14 of the 16 (87.5%) remained asymptomatic at a mean of 32.5 months after surgery (although 2 patients required a second release before becoming asymptomatic).

Conclusion

Hip bursitis are a relatively common source of hip symptoms presenting to the orthopedic surgeon. Improved knowledge regarding the functional anatomy about the greater trochanter has been obtained through advances in diagnostic imaging tools and from recent experience with hip arthroscopy. Components of this pathology include coxa saltans, trochanteric bursitis and tears of the gluteus medius and minimus.

Understanding of the common presentation and knowledge of clinical and imaging evaluation of GTPS will enable the physician to sort through the broad differential diagnosis.

In most cases the disorder is self-limiting, with treatment consisting of conservative measures such as behaviour modification, physical therapy, weight loss, and nonsteroidal anti-inflammatory drugs. When these interventions fail, bursa injections with local administration of a mixture of corticosteroid and local anaesthetic have been shown to provide good pain relief.

Endoscopic bursectomy appears to be an effective option for recalcitrant trochanteric bursitis and is a viable alternative to open bursectomy.

Because hip bursitis are so common and fairly responsive to treatment, it is important for health care providers to include this diagnosis in their differential diagnosis when evaluating hip pain.

References

[1] Voos JE, Rudzki JR, Shindle MK et al., Arthroscopic anatomy and surgical techniques for peritrochanteric space disorders in the hip. *Arthroscopy* 2007;23:1246 e1–5.

[2] Rompe JD, Decking J, Schoellner C et al., Repetitive low-energy shock wave treatment for chronic lateral epicondylitis in tennis players. *Am J Sports Med* 2004;32:734–43.

[3] Strauss EJ, Nho SJ, Kelly BT. Greater trochanteric pain syndrome. *Sports Med Arthrosc* 2010;18:113–9.

[4] Alvarez-Nemegyei J, Canoso JJ. Evidence-based soft tissue rheumatology: III: trochanteric bursitis. *J Clin Rheumatol* 2004;10:123–4.

[5] Stegemann H. Die chirurgische bedevtung paraartikularer kalkablagerungen. *Arch. Klin. Chir.* 1923; 125:718-38.

[6] Vogel WH, Berke A. Brief History of Vision and Ocular Medicine. NM Amsterdam (the Netherlands): *Kugler Publications;* 2009. p. 97.

[7] Leonard MH. Trochanteric syndrome; calcareous and noncalcareous tendonitis and bursitis about the trochanter major. *J. Am. Med. Assoc.* 1958; 168:175-7.

[8] Tortolani PJ, Carbone JJ, Quartararo LG. Greater trochanteric pain syndrome in patients referred to orthopedic spine specialists. *Spine J.* 2002; 2:251-4.

[9] Segal NA, Felson DT, Torner JC et al., Greater trochanteric pain syndrome: epidemiology and associated factors. *Arch Phys Med Rehabil* 2007;88:988–92.

[10] Williams BS, Cohen SP. Greater trochanteric pain syndrome: a review of anatomy, diagnosis and treatment. *Anesth Analg* 2009;108:1662–70.

[11] Lievense A, Bierma-Zeinstra S, Schouten B et al., Prognosis of trochanteric pain in primary care. *Br J Gen Pract* 2005;55:199–204.

[12] Swezey RL. Pseudo-radiculopathy in subacute trochanteric bursitis of the subgluteus maximus bursa. Arch Phys Med Rehabil 1976;57:387–90.

[13] Gordon EJ. Trochanteric bursitis and tendinitis. *Clin Orthop* 1961;20:193–202.

[14] Collee G, Dijkmans BA, Vandenbroucke JP et al., A clinical epidemiological study in low back pain. Description of two clinical syndromes. *Br J Rheumatol* 1990;29:354–7.

[15] Anderson K, Strickland SM, Warren R. Hip and groin injuries in athletes. *Am J Sports Med* 2001;29:521–33.

[16] Clancy WG. Runners' injuries. Part two. Evaluation and treatment of specific injuries. *Am J Sports Med* 1980;8:287–9.

[17] Schapira D, Nahir M, Scharf Y. Trochanteric bursitis: a common clinical problem. *Arch Phys Med Rehabil* 1986;67:815–7.

[18] Del Buono A, Papalia R, Khanduja V, Denaro V, Maffulli N. Management of the greater trochanteric pain syndrome: a systematic review. *British Medical Bulletin* 2012; 102: 115–131.

[19] Dunn T, Heller CA, Mc Carthy SW, Dos Remedios C. Anatomical study of the "trochanteric bursa." *Clin Anat* 2003; 16: 233–40.

[20] Margo K, Drezner J, Motzkin D. Evaluation and management of hip pain: an algorithmic approach. *J Fam Pract* 2003;52:607–17.

[21] Robertson WJ, Gardner MJ, Barker JU, et al., Anatomy and dimensions of the gluteus medius tendon insertion. *Arthroscopy.* 2008;24:130–136.

[22] Beck M, Sledge JB, Gautier E, et al., The anatomy and function of the gluteus minimus muscle. *J Bone Joint Surg Br.* 2000; 82:358–363.

[23] Birnbaum K, Siebert CH, Pandorf T, Schopphoff E, Prescher A, Niethard FU. Anatomical and biomechanical investigations of the iliotibial tract. *Surg Radiol Anat.* 2004;26:433–46.

[24] Stern Jr JT. Anatomical and functional specialization of gluteus maximus. *Am J Phys Anthropol.* 1972;36:315–39.

[25] Janecki CJ. The gluteus maximus femoral insertion: a guide in surgery about the hip. *Clin Orthop Relat Res*. 1977;123:16–8.

[26] Flack NA, Nicholson HD, Woodley SJ. A review of the anatomy of the hip abductor muscles, gluteus medius, gluteus minimus, and tensor fascia lata. *Clin Anat*. 2012;25:697–708.

[27] Apaydin N, Kendir S, Loukas M, Tubbs RS, Bozkurt M. Surgical anatomy of the superior gluteal nerve and landmarks for its localization during minimally invasive approaches to the hip. *Clin Anat.* 2012.

[28] Genth B, Von Düring M, Von Engelhardt LV, Ludwig J, Teske W, VonSchulze-Pellengahr C. Analysis of the sensory innervations of the greater trochanter for improving the treatment of greater trochanteric pain syndrome. *Clin Anat.* 2012.

[29] Sato K, Nimura A, Yamaguchi K, Akita K. Anatomical study of the proximal origin of hamstring muscles. *J Orthop Sci.* 2012;17:614–8.

[30] Hitora T, Kawaguchi Y, Mori M, Imaizumi Y, Akisue T, Sasaki K, et al., Ischiogluteal bursitis: a report of three cases with MR findings. *Rheumatol Int.* 2009;29:455–8.

[31] Ranawat AS, Kelly BT. Anatomy of the hip: open and arthroscopic structure and function. *Oper Tech Orthop.* 2005; 15:160–17.

[32] Little H. Trochanteric bursitis: a common cause of pelvic girdle pain. *Can Med Assoc J* 1979;120:456–8

[33] Shbeeb MI, Matteson EL. Trochanteric bursitis (greater trochanter pain syndrome). *Mayo Clin Proc* 1996;71:565–9.

[34] Jones DL, Erhard RE. Diagnosis of trochanteric bursitis versus femoral neck stress fracture. *Phys Ther* 1997;77:58–67.

[35] Abdelwahab IF, Bianchi S, Martinoli C, Klein M, Hermann G. Atypical extraspinal musculoskeletal tuberculosis in immunocompetent patients: part II, tuberculous myositis, tuberculous bursitis, and tuberculous tenosynovites. *Can Assoc Radiol J* 2006;57:278–86

[36] Butcher JD, Salzman KL, Lillegard WA. Lower extremity bursitis. *Am Fam Physician* 1996;53:2317–24

[37] Mandell BF. Avascular necrosis of the femoral head presenting as trochanteric bursitis. *Ann Rheum Dis 1990*;49:730–2.

[38] Silva F, Adams T, Feinstein J, Arroyo RA. Trochanteric bursitis: refuting the myth of inflammation. *J Clin Rheumatol* 2008;14:82–6.

[39] Pfirrmann CW, Chung CB, Theumann NH, Trudell DJ, Resnick D. Greater trochanter of the hip: attachment of the abductor mechanism and a complex of three bursae–MR imaging and MR bursography in cadavers and MR imaging in asymptomatic volunteers. *Radiology* 2001;221:469–77.

[40] Bunker TD, Esler CN, Leach WJ. Rotator-cuff tear of the hip. *J Bone Joint Surg Br.* 1997; 79:618-20.

[41] Kingzett-Taylor A, Tirman P, Feller J, et al., Tendinosis and tears of gluteus medius and minimus muscles as a cause of hip pain: MR imaging findings. *AJR Am. J. Roentgenol.* 1999; 173:1123-6.
[42] Lievense A, Bierma-Zeinstra S, Schouten B, et al., Prognosis of trochanteric pain in primary care. *Br. J. Gen. Pract.* 2005; 55:199-204.
[43] Tibor LM, Sekiya JK. Differential diagnosis of pain around the hip joint. *Arthroscopy* 2008;24(12):1407-21.
[44] Cohen SP, Raja SN. Pathogenesis, diagnosis, and treatment of lumbar zygapophysial (facet) joint pain. *Anesthesiology* 2007;106:591–614.
[45] Cohen SP. Sacroiliac joint pain: a comprehensive review of anatomy, diagnosis, and treatment. *Anesth Analg* 2005;101:1440–53.
[46] Ohnmeiss DD, Vanharanta H, Ekholm J. Relation between pain location and disc pathology: a study of pain drawings and CT/discography. *Clin J Pain 1*999;15:210–17.
[47] Rowand M, Chambliss ML, Mackler L. Clinical inquiries. How should you treat trochanteric bursitis? *J Fam Pract.* 2009;58(9):494-500.
[48] Rasmussen KJE, Fano N. Trochanteric bursitis. Treatment by corticosteroid injection. *Scand J Rheumatol.* 1985;14:417–420.
[49] Lequesne M. From “periarthritis” to hip “rotator cuff” tears. Trochanteric tendinobursitis. *Joint Bone Spine*. 2006;73:344–348.
[50] Lequesne M, Mathieu P, Vuillemin-Bodaghi V, Bard H, Djian P. Gluteal tendinopathy in refractory greater trochanter pain syndrome: diagnostic value of two clinical tests. *Arthritis Rheum.* 2008; 59:241-6.
[51] Adkins SB 3rd, Figler RA. Hip pain in athletes. *Am Fam Physician* 2000.1;61(7):2109-18.
[52] Bird PA, Oakley SP, Shnier R, Kirkham BW. Prospective evaluation of magnetic resonance imaging and physical examination findings in patients with greater trochanteric pain syndrome. *Arthritis Rheum.* 2001; 44:2138-45.
[53] McMahon S, Smith TO, Hing CB. A Systematic Review of Imaging Modalities in the Diagnosis of Greater Trochanteric Pain Syndrome. Musculoskelet. *Care* 2012;10:232–239.
[54] Looner JH, van Kleunen JP (2002). Spontaneous rupture of the gluteus medius andminimus tendon. *The American Journal of Orthopedics* 2002;31:579–81.
[55] Walsh G, Archibald CG.MRI in greater trochanteric pain sydrome. *Australasian Radiology* 2003;47: 85–7.
[56] Fearon AM, Scarvell JM, Cook JL, Smith PN. Does ultrasound correlate with surgical or histologic findings in greater trochanteric pain

syndrome? A pilot study. *Clinical Orthopaedics and Related Research* 2010;468:1838–44.

[57] Chung CB, Robertson JE, Cho GJ, Vaughan LM, Copp SN, Resnick D. Gluteus medius tendon tears and avulsive injuries in elderly women: Imaging findings in six patients. *American Journal of Roentgenology* 1999;173: 351–3.

[58] Cvitanic O, Henzie G, Skezas N, Lyons J, Minter. MRI diagnosis of tears of the hip abductor tendons (gluteus medius and gluteus minimus). *American Journal of Roentgenology* 2004;182: 137–43.

[59] Blankenbaker DG, Ullrick SR, Davis KW, De Smet AA, Haaland B, Fine JP. Correlation of MRI findings with clinical findings of trochanteric pain syndrome. *Skeletal Radiology* 2008;37: 903–9.

[60] Woodley SJ, Nicholson HD, Livingstone V, Doyle TC, Meikle GR, Macintosh JE, Mercer SR. Lateral hip pain: Findings from magnetic resonance imaging and clinical examination. *The Journal of Orthopaedic and Sports Physical Therapy* 2008;38: 313–28.

[61] Walker P, Kannangara S, Bruce WJ, Michael D, Van der Wall H. Lateral hip pain: Does imaging predict response to localized injection? Clinical Orthopaedics and Related Research 2007;457: 144–9.

[62] Steinert L, Zanetti M, Hodler J, Pfirrmann CW, Dora C, Saupe N. Are radiographic trochanteric surface irregularities associated with abductior tendon abdnormalities. *Radiology* 2010;257: 754–63.

[63] Berquist TH, Bender CE, Maus TP, et al., Pseudobursae: a useful finding in patients with painful hip arthroplasty. *Am J Roentgenol* 1987.148(1):103-6.

[64] Crevenna R, Kéilani M, Wiesinger G, et al., Calcific trochanteric bursitis: resolution of calcifications and clinical remission with non-invasive treatment. A case report. *Wien Klin Wochenschr* 2002;114(8-9):345-8.

[65] Connell DA, Bass C, Sykes CA, Young D, Edwards E. Sonographic evaluation of gluteus medius and minimus tendinopathy. *Eur Radiol* 2003;13(6):1339–1347

[66] Kong A, Van der Vliet A, Zadow S. MRI and US of gluteal tendinopathy in greater trochanteric pain syndrome. *Eur Radiol* 2007;17 (7):1772–1783

[67] White RA, Hughes MS, Burd T, et al., A new operative approach in the correction of external coxa saltans: the snapping hip. *Am J Sports Med.* 2004;32:1504–1508.

[68] Allen WC, Cope R. Coxa saltans: the snapping hip revisited. *J Am Acad Orthop Surg*. 1995;3:303–308.

[69] Provencher MT, Hofmeister EP, Muldoon MP. The surgical treatment of external coxa saltans (the snapping hip) by Z-plasty of the iliotibial band. *Am J Sports Med*. 2004;32:470–476.

[70] Heller A. Anatomy of the trochanteric bursae [letter]. *Radiology* 2003;226(3):921; author reply 921–922.

[71] Cohen DB, Kawamura S, Ehteshami JR, Rodeo SA. Indomethacin and celecoxib inhibit rotator cuff tendon-to-bone healing. *Am. J. Sports Med.* 2006; 34:362-9.

[72] Croisier JL, Foidart-Dessalle M, Tinant F, Crielaard JM, Forthomme B. An isokinetic eccentric programme for the management of chronic lateral epicondylar tendinopathy. *Br. J. Sports Med.* 2007; 41:269-75.

[73] Jonsson P, Wahlstrom P, Ohberg L, Alfredson H. Eccentric training in chronic painful impingement syndrome of the shoulder: results of a pilot study. *Knee Surg. Sports Traumatol. Arthrosc*. 2006; 14:76-81.

[74] Mafi N, Lorentzon R, Alfredson H. Superior short-term results with eccentric calf muscle training compared to concentric training in a randomized prospective multicenter study on patients with chronic Achilles tendinosis. *Knee Surg. Sports Traumatol. Arthrosc.* 2001; 9:42-7.

[75] Peers K, Lysens R. Patellar tendinopathy in athletes: current diagnostic and therapeutic recommendations. *Sports Med*. 2005; 35:71-87.

[76] Krout RM, Anderson TP. Trochanteric bursitis: management. *Arch Phys Med Rehabil* 1959;40:8–14.

[77] Shbeeb MI, O'Duffy JD, Michet CJ Jr, O'Fallon WM, Matteson EL. Evaluation of glucocorticosteroid injection for the treatment of trochanteric bursitis. *J Rheumatol* 1996;23:2104–6.

[78] Cohen SP, Narvaez JC, Lebovits AH, Stojanovic MP. Corticosteroid injections for trochanteric bursitis: is fluoroscopy necessary? A pilot study. *Br J Anaesth* 2005;94:100–6.

[79] Karpinski MR, Piggott H. Greater trochanteric pain syndrome. A report of 15 cases. *J Bone Joint Surg Br* 1985;67:762–3.

[80] Cohen SP, Strassels SA, Foster L et al., Comparison of fluoroscopically guided and blind corticosteroid injections for greater trochanteric pain syndrome: multicentre randomised controlled trial. *BMJ* 2009;338:b1088.

[81] Fox JL. The role of arthroscopic bursectomy in the treatment of trochanteric bursitis. *Arthroscopy* 2002;18(7):E34.

[82] Furia JP, Rompe JD, Maffulli N. Low-energy extracorporeal shock wave therapy as a treatment for greater trochanteric pain syndrome. *Am. J. Sports Med.* 2009; 37:1806Y13.

[83] Rompe JD, Segal NA, Cacchio A, et al., Home training, local corticosteroid injection, or radial shock wave therapy for greater trochanter pain syndrome. *Am. J. Sports Med.* 2009; 37:1981-90.

[84] de Jonge S, de Vos RJ,Weir A, et al., One-year follow-up of platelet-rich plasma treatment in chronic Achilles tendinopathy: a double-blind randomized placebo controlled trial. *Am. J. Sports Med.* 2011; 39:1623-9.

[85] de Vos RJ, Weir A, van Schie HTM, et al., Platelet-rich plasma injection for chronic Achilles tendinopathy - a randomized controlled trial. *JAMA.* 2010; 303:144-9.

[86] Kon E, Filardo G, Delcogliano M, et al., Platelet-rich plasma: new clinical application: a pilot study for treatment of jumper's knee. *Injury.* 2009; 40:598-603.

[87] Mishra A, Pavelko T. Treatment of chronic elbow tendinosis with buffered platelet-rich plasma. *Am. J. Sports Med.* 2006; 10:1-5.

[88] Monto RR. Platelet rich plasma (PRP) effectively treats chronic Achilles tendonosis. In: American Academy of Orthopaedic Surgeons 2010 Annual Meeting; 2010 March 12: New Orleans (LA).

[89] Paoloni J, De Vos RJ, Hamilton B, et al., Platelet-rich plasma treatment for ligament and tendon injuries. *Clin. J. Sport Med.* 2011; 21:37-45.

[90] Housner JA, Jacobson JA, Misko R. Sonographically guided percutaneous needle tenotomy for the treatment of chronic tendinosis. *J. Ultrasound Med.* 2009; 28:1187-92.

[91] Slawski DP, Howard RF. Surgical management of refractory trochanteric bursitis. *Am J Sports Med.* 1997;25:86-89.

[92] Zoltan DJ, Clancy WG, Keene JS. A new operative approach to snapping hip and refractory trochanteric bursitis in athletes. *Am J Sports Med.* 1986;14:201-204.

[93] Kagan A. Rotator cuff tears of the hip. *Clin Orthop Relat Res.* 1999; 368:135-140.

[94] Craig RA, Jones DP, Oakley AP, Dunbar JD. Iliotibial band z-lengthening for refractory trochanteric bursitis (greater trochanteric hip pain syndrome). *ANZ J Surg.* 2007;77:996-998.

[95] Farr D, Selesnick H, Janecki C, Cordas D. Arthroscopic bursectomy with concomitant iliotibial band release for the treatment of recalcitrant trochanteric bursitis. *Arthroscopy.* 2007;23:905e1-905e5.

[96] Baker CL, Massie RV, Hurt WG, Savory CG. Arthroscopic bursectomy for recalcitrant trochanteric bursitis. *Arthroscopy.* 2007;23: 827-832.

[97] Aprato A, Jayasekera N, Bajwa A, Villar RN. Peri-articular diseases of the hip: emerging frontiers in arthroscopic and endoscopic treatments. *J Orthopaed Traumatol.* 2014;15:1-11

[98] Bradley DM, Dillingham MF. Bursoscopy of the trochanteric bursa. *Arthroscopy* 1998; 14:884–887.

[99] Dunbar J., Craig R. Bursectomy and Z-lenghthening for refractory trochanteric bursitis. *J Bone Joint Surg* 2006; 88(B):312.

[100] Govaert LH, van der Vis HM, Marti RK et al., Trochanteric reduction osteotomy as a treatment for refractory trochanteric bursitis. *J Bone Joint Surg Br* 2003;85:199–203.

[101] Zimmermann B, Mikolich DJ, Ho G Jr. Septic bursitis. *Semin Arthritis Rheum* 1995;24:391.

[102] Soderquist B, Hedstrom SA. Predisposing factors, bacteriology and antibiotic therapy in 35 cases of septic bursitis. *Scand J Infect Dis* 1986;18(4):305-11.

[103] Voos JE, Shindle MK, Pruett A, et al., Endoscopic repair of gluteus medius tendon tears of the hip. *Am J Sports Med.* 2009;37:743–747.

[104] Davies H, Zhaeentan S, Tavakkolizadeh A, Janes G. Surgical repair of chronic tears of the hip abductor mechanism. *Hip Int* 2009;19:372–376.

[105] Westacott DJ, Minns JI, Foguet P. The diagnostic accuracy of magnetic resonance imaging and ultrasonography in gluteal tendon tears—a systematic review. *Hip Int* 2011;21:637–645.

[106] Domb BG, Nasser RM, Botser IB. Partial-thickness tears of the gluteus medius: rationale and technique for trans-tendinous endoscopic repair. *Arthroscopy* 2010;26:1697–1705.

[107] Faraj AA, Moulton A, Sirivastava VM. Snapping iliotibial band. Report of ten cases and review of the literature. *Acta Orthop Belg* 2001;67:19–23.

[108] Fery A, Sommelet J. The snapping hip. Late results of 24 surgical cases. *Int Orthop* 1988;12:277–282.

[109] Ilizaliturri VM Jr, Martinez-Escalante FA, Chaidez PA, Camacho-Galindo J. Endoscopic iliotibial band release for external snapping hip syndrome. *Arthroscopy* 2006;22:505–510.

[110] Ilizaliturri VM Jr, Camacho-Galindo J, Evia Ramirez AN, Gonzalez Ibarra YL, McMillan S, Busconi BD. Soft tissue pathology around the hip. *Clin Sports Med* 2011;30:391–415.

[111] Brignall CG, Stainsby GD. The snapping hip. Treatment by Z-plasty. *J Bone Joint Surg Br.* 1991;73:253–254.

In: Bursitis of Major Joints
Editor: Alessandro Aprato

ISBN: 978-1-63482-295-4

Chapter IV

Bursitis Around the Knee

Francesco Atzori[1*], MD, Luigi Sabatini[1], MD, Alessandro Stucchi[1], MD, Marcello Capella[1], MD and Wael Salama[2], MD

[1] University of Torino; Department of Orthopaedics and Traumatology; San Luigi Hospital of Orbassano; Torino, Italy

[2] University of Sohag; Orthopaedic Department; Sohag University Hospital, Sohag, Egypt

Abstract

Bursitis is inflammation of bursae. Bursae are small fluid filled sacs found all over the body. They reduce the friction between two surfaces, usually muscle/tendon and bone. This allows everything to move smoothly preventing inflammation. Bursae around the knee can be classified as those around the patella and those that occur elsewhere. Sometimes, the knee bursae get damaged which can cause pain. In this pictorial essay it is described where bursae are, the three main ways in which they can be damaged and how they could be diagnosed, the most commonly encountered lesions and their imaging. In fact, it is important for both the radiologist and the orthopaedic surgeon to be familiar with

* Corresponding author: Francesco Atzori, MD; Mail: Regione Gonzole 10, 10040 Orbassano (Torino), Italy; E-mail: f_atz@libero.it.

these bursitis as a timely corrected diagnosis may prevent unnecessary treatments. All the symptoms may or may not be present, depending on the type. Finally both conservative and surgical treatments are briefly described in order to provide a useful practice guide to an orthopedic surgeon approaching to this problem.

Introduction

Knee bursitis is inflammation of a bursa located near knee joint. Each knee has many bursae; they can be classified as those around the patella and those that occur elsewhere. Bursae around the patella include the prepatellar bursa, the superficial and deep infrapatellar bursae, and the suprapatellar bursa. Bursae that are not anatomically close to the patella include the pes anserine bursa, the iliotibial bursa, the tibial and fibular collateral ligament bursae and the gastrocnemius-semimembranosus bursa. While any of these bursae can become inflamed, knee bursitis most commonly occurs over the kneecap (prepatellar bursae) or beneath the Pes anserine.

Prepatellar bursitis are common entities, with a minimum annual incidence of 10/100,000, predominantly affecting male patients (80%) aged 40–60 years. Approximately 1/3 of cases are septic (SB) and 2/3 of cases are non-septic (NSB), with substantial variations in treatment regimens internationally.

Bursitis can lead to varying degrees of swelling, warmth, tenderness, and redness in the overlying area of the knee. As compared with knee joint inflammation (arthritis), it is usually only mildly painful. It is frequently associated with increased pain when kneeling and can cause stiffness and pain with walking. Also, in contrast to problems within the knee joint, the range of motion of the knee is frequently preserved.

Anatomy

A bursa is a synovial-lined sac overlying the bony surfaces at areas of tendon friction. Bursae are located where tendons move against each other or glide over a bony surface. They are classified according to their location: subcutaneous, subfascial, subtendinous, and submucosal [1].

Bursae can also be classified as communicating or noncommunicating. When a bursa is located adjacent to a joint, the synovial membrane of the bursae may communicate with the joint. This bursa is termed a communicating bursa. Some examples are the iliopsoas bursa lateral to the hip and the gastrocnemius-semimembranosus bursa posteromedial to the knee. In certain locations, communication between the joint and the bursa is abnormal. An example is the subacromial-subdeltoid (SASD) bursa that lies superior to the rotator cuff and inferior to the acromion [2-4].

From a histological point of view they are synovium-lined structures and are usually collapsed but may often contain a small amount of synovial fluid [5].

Bursae about the knee are numerous and normally occurring. Discussing them based on anatomic location (anterior, posterior, medial, or lateral) provides a useful means of classification. (figure 1)

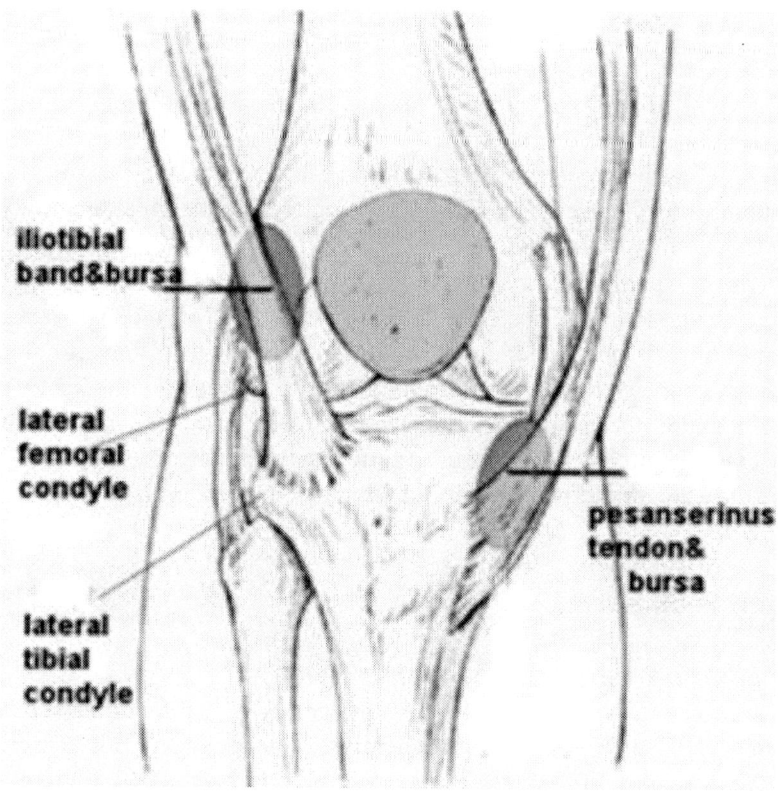

Figure 1. bursae around the knee (anteroposterior view).

Anterior Bursae

The Suprapatellar Bursa

Is a midline structure that is located between the quadriceps tendon and the femur. It normally communicates with joint, unless the suprapatellar plica, a normal embryonic septum, fails to involute, thus isolating this compartment [3].

The Prepatellar Bursa

Is located anteriorly between the patella and subcutaneous tissues. Bursitis is caused commonly by overuse injury or chronic trauma, such as occupational or recreational kneeling or crawling (housemaid's knee, carpet-layer's knee) [3].

The Superficial Infrapatellar

Also called pretibial bursa, is juxtaposed between the tibial tubercle and the overlying skin. Although this is an uncommon site of bursitis, direct trauma or occupational overuse (clergyman's knee) may result in focal inflammation or hemorrhage, causing pain anterior to the tibial tubercle [3].

The Deep Infrapatellar Bursa

Is located directly posterior to the distal third of the patellar tendon, juxtaposed between the tendon and the anterior tibia. Cadaveric study has shown no connection with the knee joint, and an average width slightly greater than the width of the distal patellar tendon. Deep infrapatellar bursitis results from extensor mechanism overuse, particularly in runners and jumpers, and manifests as anterior knee pain, mimicking patellar tendinitis [6,7].

Posterior Bursae

Semimembrnosus Gastrocnemius Bursa

Is located between the medial femoral condyle, semimembranosus tendon and the medial head of the gastrocnemius. It may or may not communicate with the knee joint [8].

The gastrocnemius-semimembranosus bursa is composed of two parts: the gastrocnemius bursa and the semimembranosus bursa. These parts may be separated partially or completely by a central septum. Depending on their intercommunication and the quantity of fluid, one or both of these structures may distend. The semimembranosus bursa is the larger of the two and is located medial to the gastrocnemius component [9].

Popliteal (Baker) Cyst

A popliteal, or Baker, cyst is the most commonly encountered cyst located about the knee. It is located in the posteromedial aspect of the knee, and represents joint fluid extending through a slit-like communication between the knee joint and the normally occurring gastrocnemius-semimembranosus bursa [10].

In 1972, Wolfe and Colloff outlined two requirements for popliteal cyst formation: an anatomic communication between the knee joint and the gastrocnemius-semimembranosus bursa, and a knee joint effusion [11,12].

Theories regarding the formation of a popliteal cyst center on the weakness of the posterior joint capsule. The posterolateral joint obtains reinforcement from the ligament of Wisberg, the popliteus tendon, and the posterior cruciate ligament (PCL) [11,12].

Conversely, the posteromedial joint has supplemental reinforcement only from the posterior horn of the medial meniscus attached to the capsule. This relative weakness, in combination with mechanical internal derangement or arthropathy, causes an increase in intra-articular pressure and a joint effusion, thus allowing joint fluid to escape through the path of lesser resistance into the gastrocnemius semimembranosus bursa [11,12].

Medial

The Pes Anserine Bursa

Is located along the medial aspect of the tibia and separates the pes anserinus, which is formed by the distal tendons of the sartorius, gracilis, semitendinosus muscles, and the distal tibial collateral ligament at the tibial insertion [3,4,9].

Pes anserine bursitis frequently results from overuse injury, often in runners, causing medial knee pain and swelling. Pes anserine bursitis commonly mimics clinically a medial meniscus tear [13].

The MCL, or Tibial Collateral Ligament Bursa

Is a vertically elongated compartment located between the superficial and deep layers of the MCL, at the level of the middle knee joint line. Cadaveric study has shown separate femoral and tibial components in most specimens [14].

The Semimembranosus-Tibial Collateral Ligament Bursa

Also located along the medial joint line, lies between the semi-membranosus tendon and the MCL, at the level of the medial tibial condyle. Inflammation may result in focal pain along the posteromedial knee at the level of the knee joint line. This bursa does not communicate with the knee joint or other medial knee bursa, although multifocal bursitis may coexist. The proximal extent of the bursa abuts the posterior horn of the medial meniscus; thus, a meniscal cyst is in the differential for a fluid collection in this location [15].

Lateral

The Iliotibial Band Bursa

Is located between the distal portion of the iliotibial band, just proximal to its insertion on Gerdy's tubercle, and the adjacent tibia. Overuse injury, commonly in runners, is the leading cause of bursal inflammation, with resultant anterolateral knee pain [3] (figure 2).

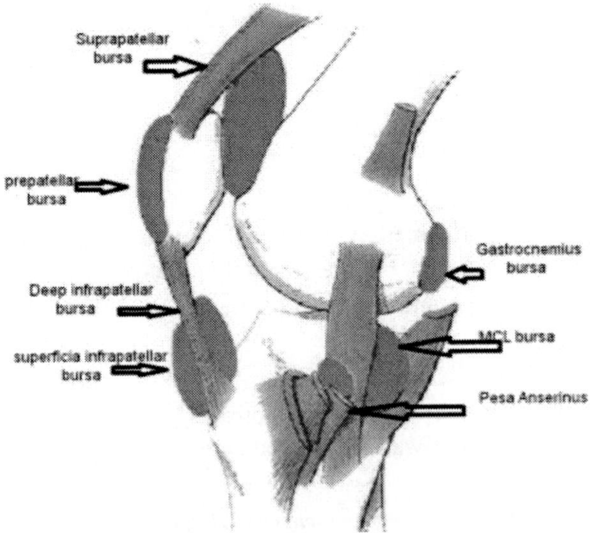

Figure 2. bursae around the knee (lateral view).

The Fibular Collateral Ligament (FCL)-Biceps Femoris Bursa

Is located lateral to the distal FCL, and extends around the anterior and anteromedial portions of this ligament. Cadaveric study has shown a consistent anatomic location, with the superior extent at the level of the crossing of the biceps femoris superficial to the FCL, and the distal extent at the insertion of the FCL on the fibular head [16].

Phisiopathology

Bursitis can develop in three main ways. It can be caused by an injury or infection, or as the result of a pre-existing health condition [17].

The predominant etiology is a traumatic lesion with or without inoculation of infectious material, mainly during professional or leisure activities Separation into septic and non-septic bursitis is possible in most cases according to clinical parameters and characteristics of the contents of the affected bursa [18].

The initial differentiation between septic (SB) and non-septic bursitis (NSB) was based on clinical presentation, bursal aspirate, and blood sampling analysis. Physical findings suggesting SB were fever >37.8 °C, prebursal temperature difference greater 2.2 °C, and skin lesions. Relevant findings for bursal aspirate were purulent aspirate, fluid-to-serum glucose ratio <50 %, white cell count >3,000 cells/μl, polymorphonuclear cells >50 %, positive Gram staining, and positive culture.

Infection

Bursae near the surface of your skin can become infected if bacteria find their way into cuts and grazes and then move into a bursa. The immune system usually prevents this type of infection, so septic bursitis tends to only occur in people with a weakened immune system. About 20% of people with knee bursitis have septic bursitis, it occurs more often in the summer months [18]. Septic bursitis usually arises from trauma resulting in direct inoculation of the bursal space. Blunt trauma, a skin wound, or repetitive pressure applied over the knee may precipitate an infection. Septic bursitis arising from infection in near by sites, such as in cases of paronychia, has also been reported. It is possible to have septic bursitis without an obvious cut or scrape; sometimes the root cause of infection is unknown. In contrast, hematogenous bacterial see ding of the bursal sac is rare, probably because of the limited vascular supply of the bursal tissue.

The population at risk for the development of septic bursitis includes laborers such as miners, gardeners, carpet layers, and mechanics, in who repetitive knee trauma is common. Those with a history of alcoholism are also prone to septic bursitis due to the repeated traumas they receive while intoxicated, coupled with their impaired host immunity. Likewise, septic bursitis has developed in some patients with impaired host defense due to the use of systemic glucocorticoids or to certain medical conditions such as malignancy, leukopenia, diabetes mellitus, or chronic renal failure. The presence of intrabursal rheumatoid nodules or gouty tophi, or a prior history of septic bursitis increases a person's risk of bursal infection. Iatrogenic sepsis may follow an intrabursal steroid injection for non septic bursitis.

Injury

If a bursa is injured, the tissue inside it can become irritated, leading to swelling.

In most cases, the injury develops over time because joints, muscles and tendons near the bursae are overused. Repetitive movement is a particular risk for this type of injury.

Ways that a bursa can be injured include:

- repeatedly moving the knee or kneeling on it
- excessive walking (particularly if not wearing suitable shoes)
- running or other impact sports
- Incorrect training techniques, or changes in terrain and/or distanced run
- Lack of flexibility in hamstring muscles
- Lack of knee extension
- Patellar malalignment

A bursa can also be injured following a sudden impact, such as falling heavily onto knees or a blunt impact in the medial aspect of them.

Health Conditions

A number of health conditions can sometimes cause a bursa to become inflamed. These include:

- gout
- rheumatoid arthritis
- scleroderma
- ankylosing spondylitis
- systemic lupus erythematosus

Traumatic and idiopathic bursitis likely have a common origin, and idiopathic cases often result from unrecognized trauma. The inciting event may be relatively trivial, such as when a person bumps the knee. The same population predisposed to septic bursitis is at risk for the development of traumatic bursitis. Chronic inflammation of prepatellar bursa after repetitive minor trauma, so called "housemaid's knee" [19], can be seen in those whose occupations require a kneeling posture, such as carpet layers and housemaids, this is the most common non septic bursitis.

The other common bursitis is the pes anserine one that is the inflammation of the bursa underlying the tendons of the sartorius, gracilis and semitendinosus (SGT) muscles [20]. These muscles provide for medial stabilization of the knee by acting as a restraint to excessive valgus opening. They also provide a counter-rotary torque function to the knee joint. The pes anserine has an eccentric role during the screw-home mechanism that dampens the effect of excessively forceful lateral rotation that may accompany terminal knee extension. Runners are affected most often. Improper training, sudden increases in distance run, and running up hills can contribute to this condition. It can also be caused by trauma such as a direct blow to this part of the knee. A contusion to this area results in an increased release of synovial fluid in the lining of the bursa. The bursa then becomes inflamed and tender or painful. Pes anserine bursitis can occur at any age, but is common in middle-aged women with knee osteoarthritis [21]. Anyone with osteoarthritis of the knee is also at increased risk for this condition. And alignment of the lower extremity can be a risk factor for some individuals. The *genu valgum* or a flatfoot position can lead to pes anserine bursitis.

The other causes of knee bursitis include infection or low-grade inflammatory conditions, such as gout, syphilis, tuberculosis, or rheumatoid arthritis. Crystal-induced bursitis most often occurs in patients with a history of gout. A minor bursal trauma may be a precipitating factor by causing intrabursal crystal shedding. Although seen infrequently, a case of calcium pyrophosphate crystal-induced bursitis from localized chondrocalcinosis may produce similar features. Finally, rheumatoid arthritis may be associated with non septic knee bursitis. Intrabursal rheumatoid nodules are occasionally present.

Clinical Evaluation

Inflammation from local and systemic processes such as overuse, trauma, internal joint derangement, inflammatory arthropathy, and collagen vascular diseases, in addition to infection and hemorrhage, may cause thickening of the synovial lining and fluid accumulation [3,4].

Bursitis can lead to varying degrees of swelling, warmth, tenderness, and redness in the overlying area of the knee. As compared with knee joint inflammation (arthritis), it is usually only mildly painful. It is frequently associated with increased pain when kneeling and can cause stiffness and pain with walking. Also, in contrast to problems within the knee joint, the range of motion of the knee is frequently preserved [3,4].

Suprapatellar Bursitis

The suprapatellar bursa extends superiorly from beneath the patella under the quadriceps femoris muscle. The patient with suprapatellar bursitis frequently has pain in the anterior knee above the patella, which can radiate superiorly into the distal anterior thigh [22]. Often, the patient is unable to kneel or walk down stairs. The patient may also have a sharp, catching sensation with range of motion of the knee, especially on first arising. Suprapatellar bursitis often coexists with arthritis and tendinitis of the knee joint, and these other pathologic processes may confuse the clinical picture [23].

Physical examination may reveal point tenderness in the anterior knee just above the patella. Passive flexion and active resisted extension of the knee reproduce the pain. Sudden release of resistance during this maneuver markedly increases the pain. Swelling in the suprapatellar region with a boggy feeling to palpation may be seen. Occasionally, the suprapatellar bursa may become infected, as evidenced by systemic symptoms including fever and malaise and local signs of rubor, color, and dolor [24].

Prepatellar Bursitis

Prepatellar bursitis is an inflammation of the prepatellar bursa which is located in front of knee. It is also called as Carpet Layer's Knee or Housemaid's Knee. This condition can develop either due to pressure or a direct injury to the knee.

Prepatellar bursitis causes pain and swelling in the area in front of the kneecap and just below. It may be very difficult to kneel down and put the knee on the floor due to the tenderness and swelling. If the condition has been present for some time, small lumps may be felt underneath the skin over the patella. Sometimes these lumps feel as though something is floating around in front of the patella, and they can be very tender. Finally, if the bursa becomes infected, the front of the knee becomes swollen and very tender and warm to the touch around the bursa anf fever can occurs. An abscess, or area of pus, may form on the front of the knee. If the infection is not treated quickly, the abscess may even begin to drain.

The Superficial Infrapatellar Bursa

The superficial infrapatellar bursa is vulnerable to injury from both acute trauma and repeated microtrauma. Superficial infrapatellar bursitis may also result from jobs that require crawling on the knees, such as laying carpet or scrubbing floors. If the inflammation of the superficial infrapatellar bursa becomes chronic, calcification of the bursa may occur [24,25].

The patient with superficial infrapatellar bursitis frequently has pain and swelling in the anterior knee over the patella that can radiate superiorly and inferiorly into the area surrounding the knee. Often, the patient is unable to kneel or walk down stairs. The patient may also have a sharp, catching sensation with range of motion of the knee, especially on first arising. Superficial infrapatellar bursitis often coexists with arthritis and tendinitis of the knee joint, and these other pathologic processes may confuse the clinical picture [25].

Deep Infrapatellar Bursitis

It most commonly results from overuse of the knee extensor mechanism, particularly in runners and jumpers. It has also been identified in patients with Osgood–Schlatter disease [26,27]. Involvement of the deep infrapatellar bursa in systemic diseases is rare [27]. Inflammation of the deep infrapatellar bursa is more difficult to detect compared to the subcutaneous bursae because of its location posterior to the patellar tendon. Clinically, the patient with deep infrapatellar bursitis exhibits pain with flexion and extension at the extremes of the range of motion. Swelling or edema is located on both sides of the patellar tendon with localized tenderness. There is no associated swelling of the patellar tendon. There may or may not be an associated knee effusion.

Popliteal (Baker) Cyst

A popliteal, or Baker, cyst is the most commonly encountered cyst located about the knee. Patients with Baker's cysts have a feeling of fullness behind the knee. Often, they notice a lump behind the knee that becomes more apparent when they flex the affected knee . The cyst may continue to enlarge and may dissect inferiorly into the calf . Occasionally, the dissection may be so significant as to cause a lower extremity compartment syndrome [28]. The pain associated with dissection into the calf may be confused with thrombophlebitis and inappropriately treated with anticoagulants. The pain of ruptured Baker's cyst that has been misdiagnosed as thrombophlebitis has been called pseudothrombophlebitis. On physical examination, the patient with Baker's cyst has a cystic swelling in the medial aspect of the popliteal fossa. Baker's cysts can become quite large, especially in patients with rheumatoid arthritis. Activity, including squatting or walking, makes the pain of Baker's cyst worse; rest and heat provide some relief. The pain is constant, is characterized as aching, and may interfere with sleep. Baker's cyst may spontaneously rupture, and rubor and color in the calf may mimic thrombophlebitis. Homan's sign is negative, and no cords are palpable [29] (Figure 3).

Pes Anserine Bursitis

Patients with pes anserine bursitis present with pain over the medial knee joint and increased pain on passive valgus and external rotation of the knee. Activity, especially involving flexion and external rotation of the knee, makes the pain worse, with rest and heat providing some relief. Often, the patient is unable to kneel or walk down stairs. Physical examination may reveal point tenderness in the anterior knee just below the medial knee joint at the tendinous insertion of the pes anserine. Swelling and fluid accumulation surrounding the bursa are often present. Active resisted flexion of the knee reproduces the pain. Sudden release of resistance during this maneuver markedly increases the pain. Rarely, the pes anserine bursa becomes infected in a manner analogous to infection of the prepatellar bursa (Figure 4).

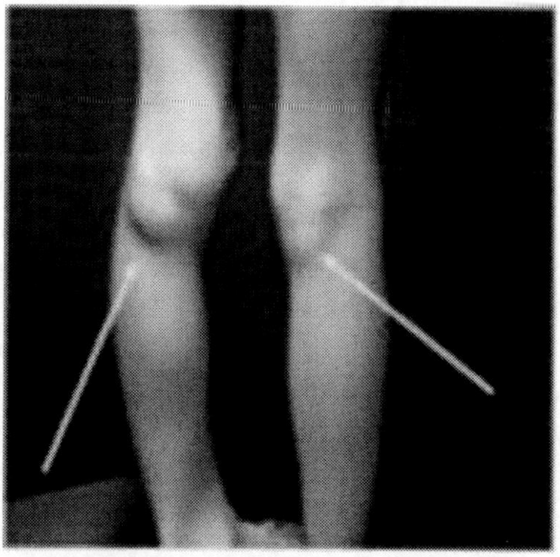

Figure 3. Bilateral Baker cysts.

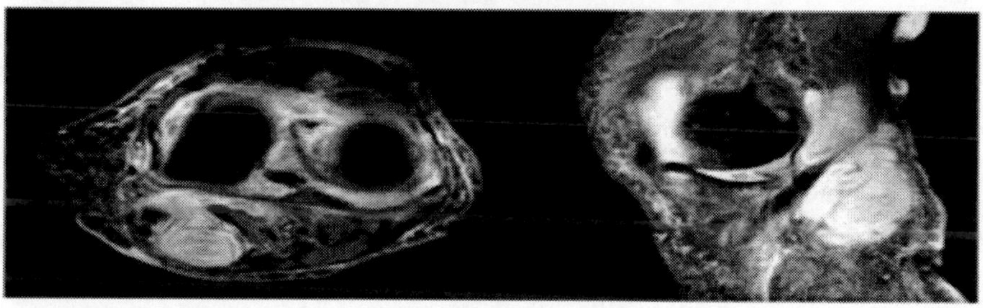

Figure 4. Baker cysts (MRI view).

Medial Collateral Ligament (MCL) Bursitis

The MCL bursa has been identified as a fluid collection between the superficial and deep MCL portions on MRIs in patients with and without (very rare) medial knee pain [30].

Clinical findings of MCL bursitis include medial knee pain and the presence of a palpable swelling along the anterior edge of the femoral portion of the MCL. The pain may be increased by applying valgus stress to the knee. The pain should be differentiated from other more common medial side conditions such as meniscal tears [31].

Fibular Collateral Ligament (FCL)-Biceps Femoris Bursa

The universal complaint associated with this bursitis is pain on the outer side of the knee. It ranges from "aching" and "burning" to "knifelike" and "stabbing" in quality. It is aggravated by exercise and, in most cases, is relieved by rest. Inspection may reveal a well-localized swelling at the joint line, varying from 0.5 to 3 centimeters in size. There is no evidence of intra-articular effusion. Upon palpation, the mass may be semi-fluctuant or firm in character ; it is not freely movable, and is tender. Tenderness is specific, and is confined to a small area at the joint line, or just inferior to it. In the cases in which no mass is evident, time tenderness is elicited by pressure on the ligament as it crosses the areas mentioned. Adduction of the extended tibia on the femur produces the pain. Combination of internal rotation and knee flexion will also produce pain in most cases [32].

Semimembranosus-Tibial Collateral Ligament Bursa

The clinical presentation is usually medial knee pain and tenderness, which can be acute or chronic. The symptoms can subside with conservative treatment and rest. The symptoms can mimic others internal derangements, the pain and tenderness usually do not occur at the expected site of pes anserinus bursa but more superiorly, posteriorly and closer to the joint line. Thus a clinician who is unaware of this newly described entity may be inclined to attribute the physical findings to a more serious cause, which may lead to unnecessary arthroscopy [33].

Imaging

Popliteal (Baker's) Cyst

Ultrasound (US) is the first-line imaging technique to investigate the presence, the localization and extent of a popliteal cyst.

The normal bursa is seen on US as a slit-like hypoechoic collection with a peripheric hyperechoic lining. The central hypoechoic part is less than 2 mm of width in healthy subjects [34]. The inferior aspect typically has a rounded configuration, with sharp appearance raising suspicion of rupture [35,36].

In rheumatoid arthritis and other inflammatory conditions, synovial proliferation and lining thickening can be observed. Echogenic material within the hypoechoic mass may suggest hemorrhagic, inflammatory or infectious etiologies [37].

Doppler can aid in the differential diagnosis between small popliteal cysts and aneurysms of the popliteal artery [37].

On magnetic resonance (MR) imaging, popliteal cysts are usually well defined and unilocular, extending posteriorly into the gastrocnemius–semimembranosus bursa, between the tendon of semimembranosus and the medial head of gastrocnemius. The gastrocnemius–semimembranosus bursa is situated along the medial side of the popliteal fossa, posterior to the upper portion of the medial femoral condyle and superficial to the medial gastrocnemius muscle [38].

In axial view, fluid can be seen wrapping around the medial gastrocnemius tendon, concave towards the midline. In smaller cysts, a septum separating the semimembranosus and the gastrocnemius components may be found [39,40].

The subgastrocnemius bursa, deep to the medial gastrocnemius muscle, is the point of communication with the posterior joint capsule and the gastrocnemius–semimembranosus bursa; it can be individuated on MR imaging in the majority of patients with popliteal cysts [41,42].

A narrow neck connecting the popliteal cyst to the knee joint is commonly identified on axial images and is usually found just below the insertion of the medial head of gastrocnemius. Along with cyst growth, the cystic fluid may extend in any direction. Inferomedial expansion is relatively common, while extension in a lateral, proximal or intyramuscolar direction is relatively rare [39, 40].

Popliteal cyst rupture is seen as high signal intensity edema in the adjacent soft tissues and fascial planes on fat-suppressed T2-weighted sequences.

Complex cysts may be septated and may contain debris or loose bodies [39-41] (Figure 4); as they lose normal fluid signal characteristics, there may be a peripheral wall enhancement after gadolinium administration, simulating a neoplastic lesion [40]. In these cases, the location of the cyst and the communication with the gastrocnemius–semimembranosus bursa may reduce the diagnostic difficulties [40]. Synovial hyperplasia, synovial sarcoma, pigmented villonodular synovitis (PVNS) and synovial osteochondromatosis can rarely originate in popliteal cysts; in the occurrence of a solid component, a contrast-enhanced MR examination should be considered to exclude a synovial tumour rather than a popliteal cyst with debris [40].

Anserine Bursitis

On US, anserine bursitis usually appears as a hypoechoic fuild collection deep to the pes anserine tendons; in some cases, particularly in chronic bursitis, it can be multiloculated with septations. The pes anserine tendons, intimately related to the fluid component, are seen as echogenic bands coursing through the hypoechoic fluid [43].

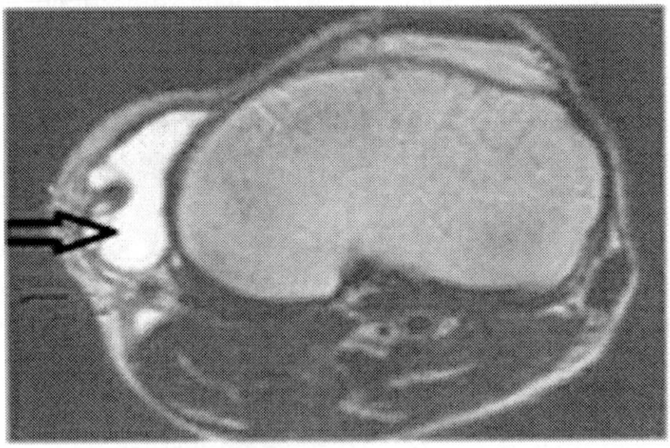

Figure 5. Pes anserine bursitis (MRI view).

On MR imaging, acute anserine bursitis appears as a homogeneous ovoid fluid superficial to the medial collateral ligament, posterior and deep to the pes anserine [38,44]. The MR appearance of chronic anserine bursitis is less specific, usually described as thickened synovial lining and fluid of heterogeneous signal intensity [38,45] (Figure5).

The differential diagnosis of acute pes anserine bursitis includes atypical synovial cysts and parameniscal cysts. The diagnosis of anserine bursitis can be made excluding a communication of the fluid collection with the knee joint and damage to the medial meniscus and the medial collateral ligament [44].

Occasional cases of giant cell tumors (extra-articular PVNS) of the anserine bursa are reported [46].

Medial Collateral Ligament Bursitis

The bursa of the medial collaterale ligament (MCL) is normally not visualized at US or MR imaging unless it is pathologically distended with fluid. This condition is typically due to medial capsuloligamentous strain or MCL tears [39,47].

MCL bursitis appears as fluid collection located between the superficial and deep portions of the MCL, vertically elongated and generally spanning the joint line on coronal view [39,47,48]. Sometimes, two distinct femoral and tibial components may be observed [48]. On axial MR images, the limits of the bursa are represented by the edge of the superficial portion of the MCL anteriorly and the junction between the superficial and deep components of the MCL posteriorly [38].

A meniscal cyst is the most realistic differential diagnosis in the case of fluid in the MCL bursa. Meniscal cysts on MR imaging demonstrate a direct communication with a meniscal tear and for this reason tend to develop in a posteromedial location [38] (Figure 6).

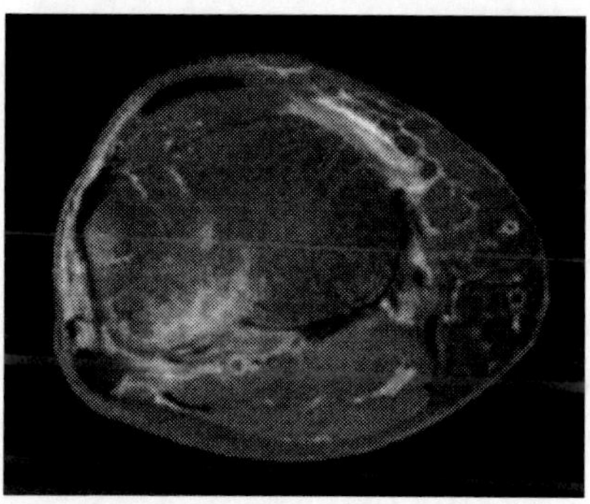

Figure 6. Chronic anserine bursitis (MRI view).

Semimembranosus–Tibial Collateral Ligament Bursitis

On MR imaging, the semimembranosus–tibial collateral ligament (SMTCL) bursitis is seen as a longitudinal fluid collection along the semimembranosus tendon, close to the medial joint line; as the semimembranosus tendon crosses the joint line posteromedially, the most proximal portion of the bursa is usually adjacent to the posterior horn of the medial meniscus [38] (figure 7).

The SMTCL bursa is located between the more superior and posterior gastrocnemius–semimembranosus bursa and the more inferior and anterior pes anserine bursa. The bursa typically drapes over the semimembranosus tendon: on axial images the bursa has the shape of an inverted U, while on coronal images it has a semilunar configuration, surrounding the tendon at its superior, medial and inferior aspect [38].

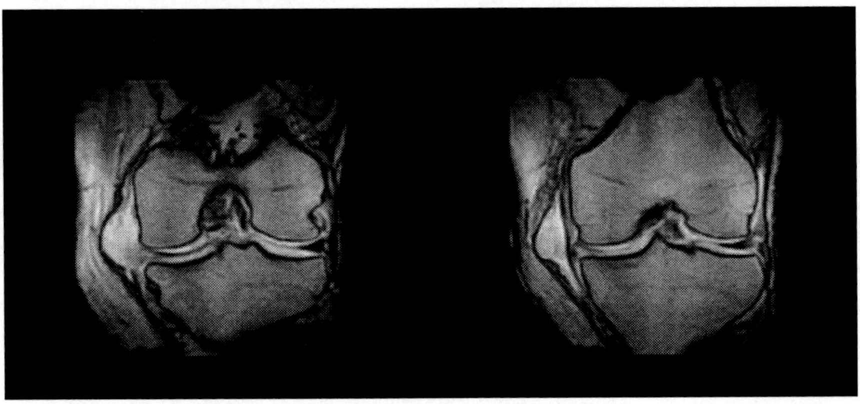

Figure 7. Medial meniscal cyst mimicking a MCL bursitis.

Prepatellar Bursitis

Fluid within the tissues anterior to the patellar tendon is frequently observed on knee MR images. Some authors consider significant a fluid thickness equal to that of the adjacent patellar tendon [38].

On MR imaging, prepatellar bursitis is seen as a fluid collection anterior to the patella and the superior part of the patellar tendon. Not infrequently, this bursa may appear poorly defined, septated or with heterogeneous signal intensity and internal debris, due to inflammation or haemorrhage. Swelling and high signal intensity edema on T2-weighted sequences may be seen in the adjacent subcutaneous fat [39].

Superficial Infrapatellar Bursitis

The small superficial infrapatellar bursa is normally not visualized on ultrasound in healthy subjects [35,37].

MR imaging may show a focal collection of fluid anterior to the tibial tubercle, best demonstrated on sagittal or axial images [38].

Deep Infrapatellar Bursitis

The deep infrapatellar bursa is located between the distal portion patellar tendon and the anterior aspect of the tibia, beneath the Hoffa's fat pad

On US, a small physiologic amount of fluid posterior to the distal patellar tendon insertion can be found [37].

On T2- weighted MR images a small amount of fluid in the deep infrapatellar bursa is occasionally seen in asymptomatic individuals; up to 2–3 mm of fluid in this bursa is considered a normal finding without clinical significance [38,39].

Suprapatellar Bursitis

The normal suprapatellar bursa can contain a small amount of physiologic fluid; US comparison with the other side is often useful in recognizing abnormally increased amounts [37]

Suprapatellar bursitis is seen on MR imaging as a focal fluid collection anterior to the distal femoral diaphysis, separated from the knee joint by a thin suprapatellar plica [39]. With chronic post-traumatic bursitis, the more heterogeneous MR signal may mimic PVNS, synovial haemangioma or synovial sarcomA [39].

Iliotibial Bursitis

Iliotibial bursitis is seen on MR imaging as a well-defined fluid collection between the insertion of the distal iliotibial band and the anterolateral aspect of the tibia. The iliotibial band syndrome, which has similar clinical features, can be differentiated on MR imaging by the presence of ill-defined high signal within the tendon on T2-weighted and STIR images [3].

Fibular Collateral Ligament–Biceps Femoris Bursitis

The fibular collateral ligament (FCL)–biceps femoris bursa is seen on MR in the axial plane as an inverted J shape around the FCL; the long arm of the J lays on the lateral aspect of the FCL, with the hook curving around the anterior edge of the FCL [5]. The distal aspect of the bursa is located just proximal to the insertion of the FCL onto the fibular head. The more proximal aspect usually correspond to the superior edge of the anterior arm of the biceps femoris muscle [50].

Conservative Treatment

As explained in previous chapters, many bursae are located around the knee. These synovially lined structures function to dampen friction between ligaments, tendons, and bone during normal knee movement. It is important for both the radiologist and the orthopaedic surgeon to be familiar with the bursae located about the knee, as bursitis may be treated conservatively in many cases, and a timely diagnosis may prevent unnecessary arthroscopy or open surgery.

For their treatment it is important to note that bursae are lined by synovium and, as a result, may be affected also by the same pathology affecting the synovium within the joint. Commonly seen pathology involving the synovium, includes rheumatoid arthritis, pigmented villonodular synovitis, and synovial osteochondromatosis. The treatment of this form is at first time the same of main pathologies with systemic use of corticosteroids; in case of uncertain diagnosis or failure of conservative treatment, surgery is then indicated.

However in most cases, when inflammation occurs, as with overuse, trauma, infection, hemorrhage, internal joint derangement, inflammatory arthropathy, or collagen vascular disease, the synovial lining may thicken, and fluid will often accumulate. Overuse and direct trauma are the chief factors that cause acute inflammatory bursitis, which may be treated with ice, rest, and nonsteroidal anti-inflammatory medications. Chronic bursitis may be treated with aspiration and local anesthetic and/or corticosteroid injections (Figure 8).

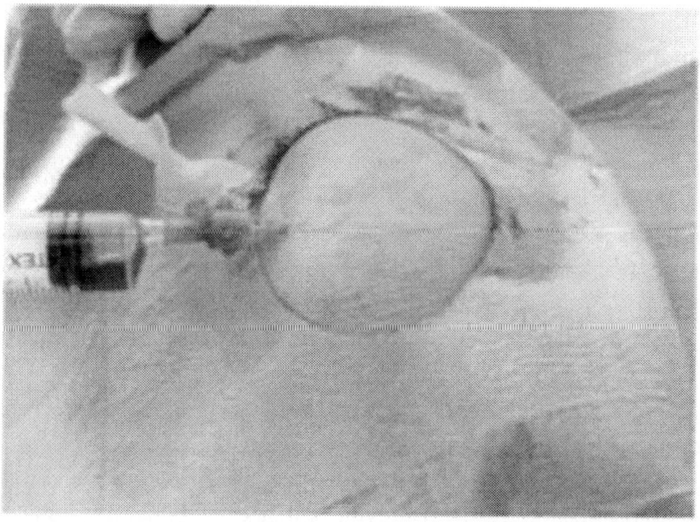

Figure 8. Bursitis aspiration.

Treatment for infectious bursitis is conservative with antibiotic therapy at the first time and drainage only for the cronic one. Other Authors suggest immediately drainage and antibiotics for infectious bursitis [51].

Traumatic lesion (acute or chronic trauma as in occupational or recreational activities) with or without inoculation of infectious material is the predominant etiology for the most common types, prepatellar and infrapatellar bursitis, in the anterior side of the knee.

Separation into septic and non-septic bursitis is possible in most cases according to clinical parameters and characteristics of the contents of the affected bursa. General treatment measures for SB and NSB are rest, ice and NSAIDS and bursal aspiration.

For patients with confirmed NSB and high athletic or occupational demands, intrabursal steroid injection may be performed. In the case of SB, antibiotic therapy should be initiated. Surgical treatment, i.e., incision, drainage, or bursectomy, should be restricted to severe, refractory, or chronic/recurrent cases. The available evidence did not support the central European concept of immediate bursectomy in cases of SB. A conservative treatment regimen should be pursued, following bursal aspirate-based differentiation between SB and NSB [52].

For bursitis in other sites, generally most difficult to reach with aspiration and injections for their position, it can be useful sonographic guidance. In literature previous authors have described successful treatment of medial collateral ligament bursitis using "blind" (non–image-guided) steroid and anesthetic mixture injections with the patient in a seated position and the knee hanging over the examination table, in combination with a quadriceps strengthening training program. However, blind injections by physicians in other anatomic locations have been shown to have poor accuracy. So some Authors suggest use of sonographic guidance for steroid injections of MCL, procedure that provides direct visualization of the medial collateral ligament bursa and confirmation of correct injection placement, resulting in increased accuracy and more successful patient outcomes. Sonographic guidance lowers the risk of inadvertently placing the steroid mixture intra-articularly or within the medial meniscal body, adjacent ligaments, or tendons. Sonography provides an excellent choice for guidance of corticosteroid injections into the medial collateral ligament bursa [53].

Repetitive microtrauma within the pes anserinus may lead to chronic inflammation and later result in development of degenerative changes in this region. It is commonly believed that this condition is caused by chronic bursitis of the pes anserinus. However, imaging studies have confirmed that as the underlying cause of complaints only in a small percentage of cases.

Rowiki et al. demonstrated that platelet rich plasma is an effective treatment for pes anserinus pain. It produces pain relief and thus significantly improves the quality of life. The response to platelet-derived growth factors was poorer in advanced degenerative knee joint disease [54].

Surgical Treatment

The treatment of bursitis around the knee is mainly determined by the cause of bursitis and surgical treatment is usually not necessary. Rest, immobilization, physical therapy and medical treatment are usually sufficient. The surgical treatment is proposed in case of pathological changes of the bursa (infection, fibrosis, etc..). Moreover, in case of failure of conservative treatment, failure of aspiration and injection of local corticosteroids and failure of drainage for acute suppurative bursitis, the surgical treatment consists of excision of chronically infected or thickened bursae.

Treatment for *prepatellar bursitis* is determined by the cause of bursitis and by the pathological change in the bursa: operative treatment is indicated when fibrosis or synovial thickening with painful nodules fails to respond to conservative treatment or in intractable bursitis, e.g. incision and drainage in cases of acute suppurative bursitis or excision of chronically infected and thickened bursa [55]. It's possible to approach the bursa with a transverse or longitudinal incision about 4-5 cm long centered over the bursa; then, resect the bursa with scissors from subcutaneous layer and deep from the patellar aponeurosis. Preferably remove the bursa without punching it. It's important to obtain a optimal hemostasis and then the wound can be closed primarily in a usual way. Some Authors prefer using suction drainage. A long compression dressing is then applied and a period of rest is necessary for 2 weeks [56] (figure 9).

In some cases of *septic patellar bursitis* are described good results with radical bursectomy and vacuum-asisted closure therapy for 4 – 5 days [57].

In case of suspect of infection of *infrapatellar bursitis*, the bursa located between the tuberosity of the tibia and the patellar tendon can be drained through a small medial parapatellar incision avoiding articular penetration [56].

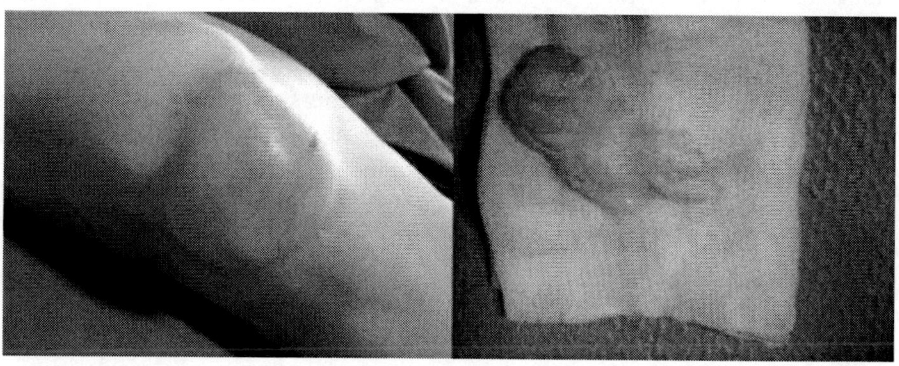

Figure 9. Prepatellar bursitis: clinical and anathomic presentation.

Iliotibial band friction sindrome is an overuse injury caused by ripetitive friction of the iliotibial band across the lateral femoral condyle. Is still controversy the nature of patological lesion responsible for the inflammatory process; for some Authors the cause is a separate bursa underlying the iliotibial band, instead for other Authors the cause is the lateral synovial recess of the knee joint. Cadaveric dissection and histological examination seem to confirm first hypothesis of a separate bursa [58].

Treatment is mostly conservative and includes rest, cold ice therapy, anti-inflammatory agents, physical therapy, local corticosteroid injection.

In rare case of patients who are not responsive to conservative management is required surgical treatment. Several surgical techiniques were reported for the treatment of iliotibial band friction syndrome: resection of a small triangular piece with base posteriorly at the posterior part of the ilitibial band covering the lateral femoral epicondyle [59] , transverse incision across the fibers of the posterior part of the iliotibial band at the level of the lateral femoral epicondyle [60], transection of the posterior half of the iliotibial band where it passed over the lateral femoral epicondyle [61], excision of an elliptical piece of the distal posterior band over the lateral femoral epicondyle [62], Z-lenghtening of the distal part of the iliotibial band [63], arthroscopic resection of the lateral synovial recess to eliminate the pain [64], multiple 2 mm long incisions spontaneously enlarged to several punctured wounds (mesh technique) across the fiber of the iliotibial band[58] and iliotibialband bursectomy without iliotibial band debridement [65].

Our surgical preference is a limited excision of the iliotibial band at the level where it passes over the most prominent part of the lateral femoral condyle with a successive bursectomy. Usually a tourniquet is inflated to 300 mm Hg; a three cm long longitudinal incision is performed over the lateral femoral condyle. The area of iliotibial band abrading the lateral femoral condyle during passive range of motion is identified and sharply incised and excised in line with its fibers. The underlying bursa is identified and excised "en bloc". Sutures of the subcutaneous layer and skin are applied in a usual way. In the postoperative time weightbearing is allowed as tolerated, usually with crutches for 1 week. Passive range of knee motion began immediatly to arrive to complete range of motion after 20-25 days. The strengthening excises of lower extremity start after 2 weeks and full returnto sport is usually possible after 3 months.

Medial collateral ligament bursitis is a rare condition of distended and inflamed bursa between the superficial and deep portions of the medial collateral ligament. Several causes have been suggested as possible causes of this type of bursitis: trauma, rheumatoid arthritis, genu valgus, osteophytosis, flatfoot deformity and friction over the medial aspect of the knee[66]. Surgical treatment is uncommon and left only to rare nonresponsive patients to conservative treatment. The surgical technique was described by Corten et al. The patient is supine with the leg if 4-figure position and a 5-cm longitudinal incision is made over the medial epicondyle. The fascia in incised from distal to the vastus medialis fibers to the insertion site of the pes anserine. The inflammatory tissue around femoral insertion of the superficial portion of the medial collateral ligament is excised in a elliptical shape and the interval between superficial and deep portions is abraded with a curette. The interval between the deep and superficial medial collateral portions is closed with horizontal absorbable stitches. The knee is immobilized in a brace fixed in 30° of flexion for 5 weeks and the weightbearing is not allowed for 3 weeks; sport activities begin after 12 weeks [66].

Fibular collateral ligament bursitis has not to be confused with a cyst of the lateral meniscus; it's extrasynovial and places beneath the fibular collateral ligament. Treatment is usually conservative with rest, cold ice therapy and local corticosteroid injection; when the bursa is palpable and symptomatic (also more than 2 cm in diameter), surgical excision is proposable by local resection with small longitudinal incision.

Pes anserine bursitis appears usually as a distended bursa on the medial side of the popliteal space on the lateral side of the semimembranosus tendon. This condition is not to confuse with anserine syndrome, a spontaneous medial knee pain with tenderness in the inferomedial aspect of the joint: diabetes mellitus, overweight and osteoarthritis are predisposing factor to this syndrome that needs conservative treatment. In case of real semimembranosus bursitis, surgical treatment can be useful in chronic cases. The patient is supine and the incision is 8.0 cm long over the medial aspect of the popliteal space, slightly oblique. After incising the deep fascia, open the interval between the semimembranosus and the medial head of the gastrocnemius; divide the cyst wall with safe dissection from the semimembranosus and the medial head of the gastrocnemius, avoiding cyst's rupture. Try to remove the bursa, or the wall in case of rupture, completely with scissors until the base on the capsule. After usual closure without drainage, the knee is immobilized for 2 weeks in light flexion.

Are also described very rare cases of extra-articular pigmented villonodular synovitis arising from the bursa (pigmented villonodular bursitis or diffuse giant cell tumor of the tendon sheath); the surgical treatment suggested is similar [67].

Medial gastrocnemius bursitis can show as a palpable mass located in the midline of the popliteal space; in this case, can be necessary a posterior incision with patient in prone position. Trickey incision is an efficient approach; dissection is carried to the deep fascial layer, wich is incised vertically over the medial head of the gastrocnemius. The medial sural cutaneous nerve has to be protected while perforates the deep fasciae in the distal part of the incision. The plane between the medial border of the medial gastrocnemius and the semimembranosus is developed by blunt dissection, until the posterior joint capsule is reached. Then, clamp the pedicle of the cyst to the capsule and divided it. Rest and elastic compression bandage is suggest for 2 weeks.

Arthroscopic Resection

Open excision of bursa around the knee can be complicated by hypoesthesia secondary to nerve damage, wound breakdown, painful scar, poor scar cosmesis, skin necrosis, infection and prolonged recovery [68].

So arthroscopic excision can be an alternative, expecially for prepatellar bursa and can be performed for both aseptic and septic prepatellar bursitis [69]. Instead some Authors, endoscopic bursectomy is a safe and effective treatment for septic pre-patellar bursitis with a shortened hospital stay and a quicker return to work than conventional open debridement [70].

Kerr and Carpenter first described arthroscopic excision of the prepatellar bursa and Ogilvie-Harris and Gilbart reported satisfactory results for endoscopic resection of prepatellar bursa [71,72].

As for traditional open resection, before starting endoscopic resection is mandatory to rule out an infectious etiology; in this case, peri-operative antibiotics are administred after than a specimen is collected for microbiological analysis. It's possible injecting cortisone into the bursa some days before surgery in non-septic cases to decrease local inflammation state. Endoscopic resection is otherwise tecnically challenging. Standard anteromedial and anterolateral superficial portals can be used, but it's important to avoid damage to infrapatellar nerve; if necessary, a superior lateral portal is also made. Before inserting the arthroscope, the bursa has to be inflated by injecting normal saline. It's possible to use a 4.5 mm curved shaver to remove all the bursal sack that could be seen and the resection should go from subcutaneous area of the skin until to fibers of the patellar tendon: it's important to avoid penetration of the shaver into superficial skin or into patellar tendon. Some Authors prefer using 2.7 mm diameter endoscope and motorised shaver[55]. The portals can be left open to allow drainage. Rest and elastic compression bandage is suggested for one week and patient can achieve normal activities after 3 – 4 weeks.

Unsatisfacory results are described in patients with an inflammatory cause of prepatellar bursitis, such as rheumatoid arthritis; complications of endoscopic resection of prepatellar bursa are superficial wound infection, delayed wound closure, recurrence of bursitis and secondary patellar tendon rupture [71,73].

Also in case of *pes anserinus bursitis* are described good results with debridement under *arthroscopy*: less complication, low relapse rate and good functional rehabilitation versus local block therapy and open surgery [74].

Popliteal cysts, meniscal cysts, proximal tibiofibular joint cysts (figure 10) and cruciate ligament ganglion cysts are *cystic masses* with different etiopatologhy than around the knee bursitis; only the Baker cysts form when a bursa swells with synovial fluid. However, in simptomatic cases, these cystic masses are managed with open or arthroscopic excision [75].

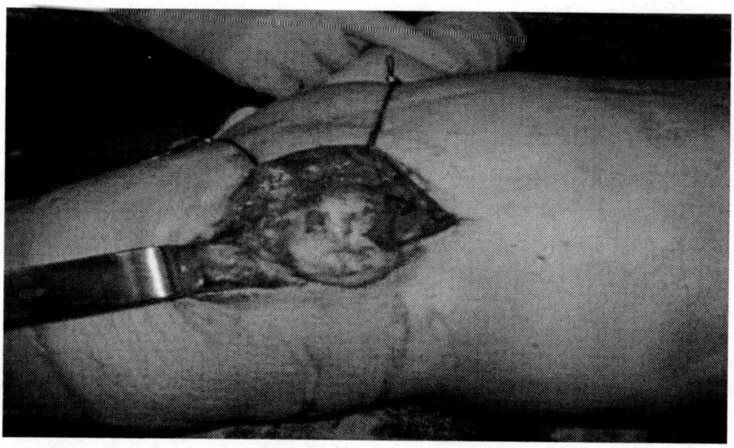

Figure 10. Proximal tibiofibular joint cyst.

References

[1] Resnick D. 3rd ed. Philadelphia (PA): W.B. Saunders; 1995. *Diagnosis of Bone and Joint Disorders;* pp. 667–8.

[2] Farooki S, Ashman C, Lee J, Guttikonda S, Yu J. Common bursae around the body: A review of normal anatomy and magnetic resonance imaging findings. *Radiologist.* 2002;9:209–11.

[3] Janzen DL, Peterfy CG, Forbes JR, et al. Cystic lesions around the knee joint: MR imaging findings. *AJR Am J Roentgenol* 1994;163:155–61.

[4] McCarthy CL, McNally EG. The MRI appearance of cystic lesions around the knee. *Skeletal Radiol* 2004;33:187–209.

[5] Evangelos Perdikakis, Vasilios Skiadas .MRI characteristics of cysts and "cyst-like" lesions in and around the knee: what the radiologist needs to know. *Insights Imaging* (2013) 4:257–272.

[6] Tschirch FTC, Schmid MR, Pfirrmann CWA, et al.Prevalence and size of meniscal cysts, ganglionic cysts, synovial cysts of the popliteal space, fluidfilled bursae, and other fluid collections in asymptomatic knees on MR imaging. *AJR Am J Roentgenol* 2003;180:1431

[7] LaPrade RF. The anatomy of the deep infrapatellar bursa of the knee. *Am J Sports Med* 1998;26:129–32.

[8] Dhillon M, Prasad P, Goel A, Kar A. Giant osteochondral body in popliteal cyst. *Indian J Orthop.* 2009;43:93–6. [PMC free article] [PubMed].

[9] Lee KR, Cox GG, Neff JR, et al. Cystic masses of the knee: arthrographic and CT evaluation. *AJRAm J Roentgenol* 1987;148:329–34.

[10] Lindgren PG, Willen R. Gastrocnemio-semimembranosus bursa and its relation to the knee joint.II. Post mortem radiography. *Acta Radiol* 1977;18:698–704.

[11] Wolfe RD, Colloff B. Popliteal cysts. An arthrographic study and review of the literature. *J Bone Joint Surg Am* 1972;54:1057–63.

[12] Labropoulos N, Shifrin DA, Paxinos O. New insights into the development of popliteal cysts. *Br J Surg* 2004;91:1313–8.

[13] Rennie WJ, Saifuddin A. Pes anserine bursitis: incidence in symptomatic knees and clinical presentation. *Skeletal Radiol* 2005;34:395–8.

[14] De Maeseneer M, Shahabpour M, Van Roy F, et al. MR imaging of the medial collateral ligament bursa: findings in patients and anatomic data derived from cadavers. *AJR Am J Roentgenol* 2001;177:911–7.

[15] Rothstein CP, Laorr A, Helmes CA, et al. Semimembranosus-tibial collateral ligament bursa:MR imaging. *AJR Am J Roentgenol* 1996;166:875–7.

[16] LaPrade RF, Hamilton CD. The fibular collateral ligament-biceps femoris bursa. An anatomic study. Am J Sports Med 1997;25:439–43

[17] Hirji Z, Hanjun JS, Choudur HN. Imaging of Bursae. *J Clin Imaging Sci.* 2011;1:22.

[18] Daniel L. Aaron, Amar Patel, Sephen Kayioros, and Ryan Calfee. "Four Common Types of Bursitis: Diagnosis and Management." *JAAOS June* 2011, vol. 19, no. 6, p. 359-367.

[19] Lee P, Hunter TB, Taljanovic M. Musculoskeletal colloquialisms: How did we come up with these names? *Radiographics*. 2004;24:1009–27.

[20] Rennie WJ, Saifuddin A. Pes anserine bursitis: Incidence in symptomatic knees and clinical presentation. *Skeletal Radiol*. 2005;34:395-398.

[21] Butcher JD, Salzman KL, Lillegard WA. Lower extremity bursitis. *Am Fam Physician*. 1996;53:2317-2324

[22] S.D. Waldman: Suprapatellar bursitis. S.D. Waldman Atlas of common pain syndromes.ed 2 2008 *Saunders Philadelphia* 309-311

[23] F.D. Beaman, J.J. Peterson: MR imaging of cysts, ganglia, and bursae about the knee. *Radiol Clin North Am*. 45:969 2007 17981178

[24] S.D. Waldman: Bursitis syndromes of the knee. S.D. Waldman Pain review. 2009 Saunders Philadelphia 318-322.

[25] S.D. Waldman: Superficial infrapatellar bursitis. S.D. Waldman Atlas of common pain syndromes. ed 2 2008 *Saunders Philadelphia* 314-315

[26] McCarthy CL, McNally EG (2004) The MRI appearance of cystic lesions around the knee. *Skeletal Radiol* 33(4):187–209

[27] Rosenberg ZS, Kawelblum M, Cheung YY, Beltran J, Lehman WB, Grant AD (1992) Osgood–Schlatter lesion: fracture or tendinitis? Scintigraphic, CT, and MR imaging features. *Radiology* 185(3):853–858

[28] Jubran T. Alqanatish , Ross E. Petty , Kristin M. Houghton , Jaime Guzman ,Lori B. Tucker, David A. Cabral ,Robyn A. Cairns Infrapatellar bursitis in children with juvenile idiopathic arthritis: a case series. *Clin Rheumatol* (2011) 30:263–267.

[29] Pain management 2nd edition , by Steven D. Waldman.

[30] Barclay C, Springgay G, van Beek E, Rolf C. Medial collateral ligament bursitis in a 12-year-old girl. *Arthroscopy*. 2005;21:759.

[31] Kerlan RK, Glousman RE. Tibial collateral ligament bursitis. *Am J Sports Med*. 1988;16:344- 346.

[32] I.E. Hendryson. Bursitis in theregion of the fibular collateral ligament. *J Bone Joint Surg Am*, 1946 Jul; 28 (3): 446-450.

[33] Christopher P, Rothstein, Alan Laorr ,Clyde A, Helms Phillip F, J. Tirman .Semimembranosus-Tibial Collateral Ligament Bursitis: MR Imaging Findings. *AJR* 1996;166:875-877.

[34] Strome GM, Bouffard JA, Van Holsbeeck M. Knee. *Clin Diagn Ultrasound 1*995; 30:201–219.

[35] Grobbelaar N, Bouffard JA. Sonography of the knee: a pictorial review. *Semin Ultrasound CT MR* 2000; 21:231–274.

[36] Ptasznik R. Ultrasound in acute and chronic knee injury. *Radiol Clin North Am* 1999; 37:797–830.

[37] Friedman L, Finlay K, Jurriaans E. Ultrasound of the knee. *Skeletal Radiol* 2001; 30:361-377.

[38] McCarthy C, McNally E: The MRI appearance of cystic lesions around the knee. *Skeletal Radiol* 2004, 33:187–209.

[39] Steiner E, Steinbach LS, Schnarkowski P, Tirman PFJ, Genant HK. Ganglia and cysts around joints. *Radiol Clin North Am* 1996; 34:400–410.

[40] Torreggiani WC, Al-Ismail K, Munk PL, et al. The imaging spectrum of Baker's (popliteal) cysts. *Clin Radiol* 2002; 57:681–691.

[41] Miller TT, Staron RB, Koenigsberg T, Levin TL, Feldman F. MR imaging of Baker cysts: association with internal derangement, effusion and degenerative arthropathy. *Radiology* 1996; 201:247– 250.

[42] Ward EE, Jacobson JA, Fessel DP, Hayes CW, Van Holsbeeck M. Sonographic detection of Baker's cysts: comparison with MR imaging. *AJR Am J Roentgenol* 2001; 176:373–380.

[43] Grover RP, Rakhra KS. Pes anserine bursitis - an extra-articular manifestation of gout. *Bull NYU Hosp Jt Dis.* 2010;68:46–50.

[44] Forbes JR, Helms CA, Janzen DL. Acute pes anserine bursitis: MR imaging. *Radiology* 1995; 194:525–527

[45] Zeiss J, Coombs R, Booth R, Saddemi S. Chronic bursitis presenting as a mass in the pes anserine bursa: MR diagnosis. *J Comput Assist Tomogr* 1993; 17:137– 140.

[46] Maheshwari AV, Muro-Cacho CA, Pitcher JD. Pigmented villonodular bursitis/diffuse giant cell tumor of the pes anserine bursa: a report of two cases and review of literature. *Knee* 2007; 14: 402–407.

[47] Lee JK, Yao L. Tibial collateral ligament bursa: MR imaging. *Radiology* 1991; 178:855–857.

[48] De Maeseneer M, Shahabpour M, Van Roy F, et al. MR imaging of the medial collateral ligament bursa: findings in patients and anatomic data derived from cadavers. *AJR Am J Roentgenol* 2001; 177:911–917.

[49] Aydingoz U, Oguz B, Aydingoz O, Comert RB, Akgun I. The deep infrapatellar bursa: prevalence and morphology on routine magnetic resonance imaging of the knee. J Comput Assist Tomogr 2004; 28: 557-561.

[50] LaPrade RF, Hamilton CD. The fibular collateral ligament–biceps femoris bursa. An anatomic study. Am J Sports Med 1997; 25:439–443

[51] Freys SM. Olecranon and pre-patellar bursitis. *Arch Chir Suppl Kongressbd.* 1997;114:493-6.

[52] Baumbach SF1, Lobo CM, Badyine I, Mutschler W, Kanz KG. Prepatellar and olecranon bursitis: literature review and development of a treatment algorithm. *Arch Orthop Trauma Surg.* 2014 Mar;134(3):359-70.

[53] Jean Jose, DO, Erica Schallert, MD, Bryson Lesniak, MD Sonographically Guided Therapeutic Injection for Primary Medial (Tibial) Collateral Bursitis *J Ultrasound Med* 2011; 30:257–261

[54] Rowicki K1, Płomiński J1, Bachta A2 Evaluation of the effectiveness of platelet rich plasma in treatment of chronic pes anserinus pain syndrome. *Ortop Traumatol Rehabil.* 2014 May-Jun;16(3):307-18.

[55] Huang YC, Yeh WL. Endoscopic treatment of prepatellar bursitis. *International Orthopaedics* 2011; 35: 355-58.

[56] Campbell's Operative Orthopaedics. Edited by S. Terry Canale, ninth edition, vol. 1, 776-82.

[57] Walter G, Kemmerer M, Hoffmann R. Treatment of septic olecranon and patellar bursitis by excision and vacuum-assisted closure therapy. *Z Orthop Unfall* 2013 Aug; 151(4):353-7.

[58] Sangkaew C. Surgical tratment of iliotibial band friction syndrome with the mesh technique. *Arch Orthop Trauma Surg* 2007; 127:303-06.

[59] Martens M, ibbrecht P, Burssens A. Surgical treatment of the iliotibial band friction syndrome. *Am J Sports Med* 1989; 17:651-54.

[60] Noble CA. The treatment of iliotibial band friction syndrome. *Am J Sports Med* 1979;13:51-54.

[61] Drogset JO, Rossvoll I, Grontvedt T. Surgical reatment of iliotibial band friction sindrome. A retrospective study of 45 patients. *Scand J Med Sci Sports* 1999; 9:296-98.

[62] Holmes JC, Pruitt AL, Whalen NJ. Iliotibial band syndrome in cyclists. *Am J Sports Med* 21;419-24.

[63] Richards DP, Barber FA, Troop RL. Iliotibial band Z-lengthening. *Arthroscopy* 2003;19:326-29.

[64] Nemeth WC, Sanders BL. The lateral synovial recess of the knee: anatomy and role in chronic iliotibial band friction syndrome. *Arthroscopy* 1996; 12:574-80.

[65] Hariri S, Savidge ET, Reinold MM, Zachazewski J, Gill T. Treatment of recalcitrant iliotibial band friction syndrome with open iliotibial band

bursectomy: indications, technique, and clinical outcomes. *Am J Sports Med* 2009;37, 7: 1417-24.
[66] Corten K, Vandenneucker H, Van Lauwe J, Bellemans J. Chronic posttraumatic bursitis of the medial collateral ligament. Surgical treatment in 2 high-level professional athletes. *Tha American Journal of Sports Medicine* 2009; 37, 3: 610-13.
[67] Maheshwari AV, Muro-CAcho CA, Pitcher JD. Pigmented villonodular bursitis/diffuse giant cell tumor of the pes anserine bursa: a report of two cases and review of literature. *The Knee* 2007; 14: 402-07.
[68] Quayle JB, Robinson MP. An operation for chronic prepatellar bursitis. *J Bone Joint Surg Br.* 1976;58:504-6.
[69] Kaalund S, Breddam M, Kristensen G. Endoscopic resection of the septic prepatellar bursa. *Arthroscopy.* 1998;14:757-8.
[70] Dillon JP, Freedman I, Tan JSM, Mitchell D, English S. Endoscopic bursectomy for the treatmnent of septic pre-patellar bursitis: a case series. *Arch Orthop Trauma Surg* 2012; 132:921-25.
[71] Kerr DR, Carpenter CW. Arthroscopic resection of olecranon and prepatellar bursae. *Arthroscopy.* 1990;6:86-8.
[72] Ogilvie-Harris DJ, Gilbart M. Endoscopic bursal resection: the olecranon bursa and prepatellar bursa. *Arthroscopy.* 2000;16:249-53.
[73] Epstein DM, Capeci CM, Rokito AS. Patella tendon rupture after arthroscopic resection of the prepatellar bursa: a case report. *Bulletin of the NYU Hospital for Joint Diseases*. 2010; 68(4): 307-10.
[74] Yan C, Chen B, Shao D, Kang H, Liu H, Wang S, Li J. *Zhongguo Xiu Chong Jian Wai Ke Za Zhi* 2009; Sep; 23(9):1045-8.
[75] Stein D, Cantlon M, Mackay B, Hoelscher C. *J Am Acad Orthop Surg* 2013 Aug; 21 (8):469-79.

In: Bursitis of Major Joints
Editor: Alessandro Aprato

ISBN: 978-1-63482-295-4

Chapter V

Bursitis Around the Ankle

Michel Calò[1], Roberto Rossi[2] and Davide Edoardo Bonasia[2,*]

[1]University of Torino Department of Orthopaedics and Traumatology AO Città della Salute e della Scienza – Torino, Italy

[2]University of Torino Department of Orthopaedics and Traumatology AO Mauriziano "Umberto I" Largo Turati – Torino, Italy

Abstract

Joint bursitis is an inflammatory disease of one of the bursae positioned around a joint. Of all ankle bursae, most authors agree that the retrocalcaneal bursa is the most frequently affected by inflammation. Multiple causes for ankle bursitis have been recognized and include an overuse of the joint, infection, direct injuries (contusions) or rheumatic diseases. Other conditions such as Haglund's deformity cause impingement between the Achilles tendon and the promiment posterosuperior calcaneal tuberosity, resulting in retrocalcanear bursitis (RB). The diagnosis begins with an accurate patient's history and physical examination. The imaging includes an x-ray study and, in order to better evaluate the soft tissues and possible inflammation, ultrasound and MRI can be used. The treatment starts with a conservative approach, however, about 15–50% of the patients suffering from chronic (more than

* Corresponding author: Davide E. Bonasia, MD Via Lamarmora 26, 10128, Torino, Italy Ph: (+39) 3356068525 Email: davidebonasia@virgilio.it.

3 months) RB do not benefit from conservative management, mostly when Haglund's deformity is present, and consequently undergo surgical treatment. Resection of the retrocalcaneal bursa and Haglund's tuberosity is the main focus of operative treatment for RB. This can be obtained either via open or endoscopy surgery. Open surgery requires large exposure with a consequent high risk of wound and soft tissue problems, especially in this anatomical area where the circulation is poor. Numerous studies and substantial progress have been made regarding arthroscopic/endoscopic ankle surgery.

Keywords: Haglund, retrocalcaneal bursitis, ankle, endoscopy

Introduction

Joint bursitis is an inflammatory disease of one of the bursae positioned around a joint. The inflammation of ankle bursae can be relatively frequent especially in athletes. Of all ankle bursae, most authors agree that the retrocalcaneal bursa is the most frequently affected by inflammation. Chronic retrocalcaneal bursitis (RB) is an inflammation of the bursa located between the Achilles tendon and the posterior border of the calcaneus. Painter made the first description of this disease in 1898 [1], and the first successful surgical treatment was performed by Haglund and described in 1928 [2]. Chronic RB was previously described with different confusing names as Haglund's deformity, pump bump, and winter heel. Recently, this condition has been defined as "chronic retrocalcaneal bursitis [3]. The goal of this chapter is to describe the anatomy, physiopathology, clinical evaluation, imaging, conservative and surgical treatments for ankle bursitis, with particular attention to the RB.

Anatomy

Several tendons, muscles, and ligaments support the ankle joint. Ankle joint bursae act as cushions between tendons, ligaments, muscles and ankle joint bones, resulting in decreased friction between these structures. Viscous fluid within bursae is produced by synovial membrane.

Within the ankle, four major bursae can be recognized (Figure 1).

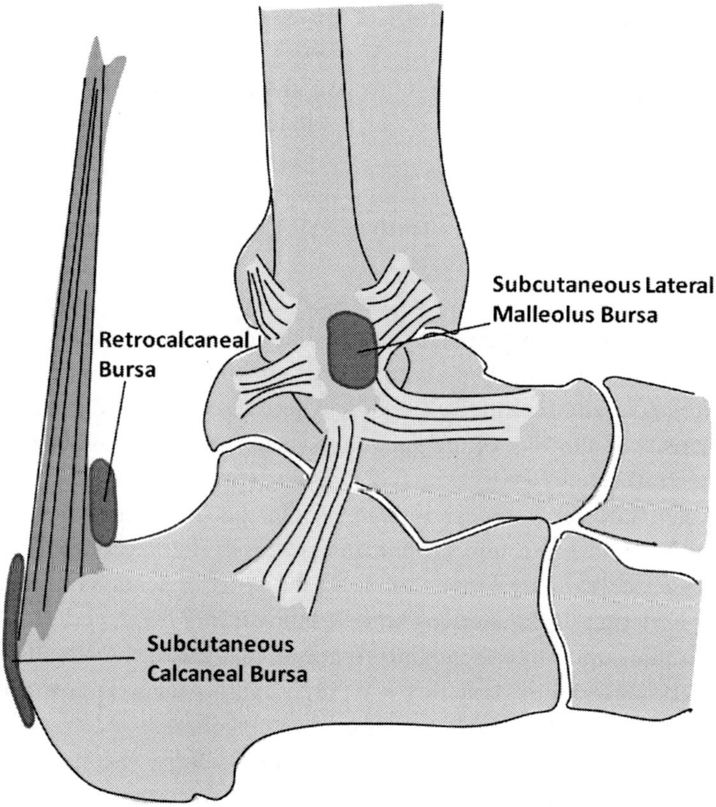

Figure 1. Lateral aspect of the ankle showing the location of the Retrocalcaneal Bursa, Subcutaneous Calcaneal Bursa, and Subcutaneous Lateral Malleolus Bursa.

Retrocalcaneal Bursa

The retrocalcaneal bursa lies between the calcaneus bone and the Achilles tendon. This bursa helps prevent injuries to Achilles tendon.

Subcutaneous Calcaneal Bursa

The subcutaneous calcaneal bursa is located between the posterior surface of calcaneal bone and the subcutaneous tissue.

Subcutaneous Medial Malleolus Bursa

This bursa is located between the skin and the medial malleolus and helps create smooth flexion/extension of the ankle joint.

Subcutaneous Lateral Malleolus Bursa

This bursa is located between the skin and the lateral malleolus and has the same function as the subcutaneous medial malleolus bursa.

In addition, tendon sheaths are modified bursae protecting the tendons from friction circumferentially, mostly where retinacula are present. On the lateral aspect of the ankle, the common sheath of the peroneus longus and brevis helps the tendons gliding behind the lateral malleolus and under the superior and inferior peroneal retinacula. On the dorsal aspect of the ankle, tendinous sheaths are found around the extensor digitorum longus/peroneus tertius, extensor hallucis longus, and tibialis anterior tendons. These sheaths reduce the friction of the tendons while gliding under the superior and inferior extensor retinacula. On the medial aspect of the ankle, the tibialis posterior, flexor digitorum longus, and flexor hallucis longus tendons are protected by individual sheaths at the level of the flexor retinaculum.

As mentioned above, the retrocalcaneal bursa is more prone to inflammation compared with the other bursae. A recent histological study showed that the retrocalcaneal bursa was constantly present in all the cadavers examined, and its volume varied from 1 to 1.5 ml [4]. The histological analysis confirmed that the inner surface of the superior and posterior wall of the retrocalcaneal bursa was covered by unilayered synovial membrane, projecting into synovial villi of different shapes and sizes. In the ceiling of retrocalcaneal bursa, a delicate fascicle of skeletal muscle fibers was identified, radiating distally into the regularly present synovial fold. A 200–500 μm layer of fibrous cartilage attached to the Achilles tendon covered the distal part of retrocalcaneal bursa. The cartilagineous layer continued anteroproximally to cover the whole bursal surface of the calcaneal tuberosity, where the thickness of the cortical bone was reduced [4]. The histopathology of the retrocalcaneal bursa included fibro-cartilaginous bursal walls showing degeneration and/or calcification, with hypertrophy of the synovial infoldings and accumulation of fluid in the bursa. Alternatively, the bursa was primarily involved by inflammatory or infectious tissue due to an inflammatory arthropathy [4].

Physiopathology

Multiple causes for ankle bursitis have been recognized. These include overuse of the ankle joint (e.g., cycling and jogging cause bursitis around the ankle joint), infection, direct injuries (contusions), or rheumatic diseases. Haglund's deformity causes impingement between the Achilles tendon and the promiment posterosuperior calcaneal tuberosity, resulting in RB. Also tight fitting shoes can cause increased pressure over the ankle joint bursae with consequent bursitis. In this last case, mostly subcutaneous bursae are involved, but also the retrocalcaneal bursa may be affected. In addition, malaligned hindfoot may result in an asymmetrical load on the Achilles tendon and altered biomechanics. This condition can be associated with an increased risk for Achilles tendon pathologies, including bursitis [5].

Clinical Evaluation

The diagnosis begins with an accurate patient's history and physical examination.

Footwear has to be investigated, such as high-heeled shoes or tight-fitting athletic shoes. Specifically, recent changes in footwear (e.g., new athletic shoes, transition from flat shoes to high heels) have to be evaluated. Patients wearing high-heeled shoes on a long-term basis may experience increased stretch and irritation of the Achilles tendon and RB. Patient's physical activity level has to be investigated (e.g., long-distance runners). Previously known or suspected underlying rheumatologic conditions (e.g., gout, rheumatoid arthritis, seronegative spondyloarthropathies) or other systemic conditions have to be considered. The diagnosis continues with an accurate physical examination. The patient with RB often reports painful swelling medial and/or lateral to the Achilles tendon. Swelling and redness of the posterior heel may also be evident. The inflamed area may be slightly warm and tender to palpation.

Accurate examination can help the physician to distinguish whether the inflammation is posterior to the Achilles tendon (superficial, within the subcutaneous bursa) or anterior to the Achilles tendon (deep, within the subtendinous bursa). Tenderness caused by RB can best be elicited by palpation just anterior to both the medial and lateral edges of the distal Achilles tendon.

Differential diagnoses for RB include: 1) Sever's Disease (in children or young adolescents); 2) Plantar fasciitis; 3) Achilles tendonitis; 4) partial rupture of the Achilles tendon; 5) Calcaneal stress fractures; 6) Tarsal coalitions; 7) Nerve entrapment symdromes; 8) Tumors (Osteoid osteoma, Osteochondroma, Chondroblastoma, Bone cyst, leukemia); 9) Infection – abscess, osteomyelitis; 10) Calcaneal exostosis; 11) Contusion; 12) Heel fat pad syndrome; 13) Posterior ankle impingement/flexor hallucis longus tendonitis; and 14) Rheumatic arthropathies.

Tenderness due to insertional Achilles tendonitis is located slightly more distal, where the Achilles tendon inserts onto the posterior calcaneus. Plantar fasciitis causes tenderness along the posterior aspect of the sole, and patients should not experience tenderness with palpation of the posterior heel or ankle. A patient with avulsion or rupture of the Achilles tendon shows a palpable defect in the tendon and a positive Thompson test, but only if the tear is complete.

Subcutaneous bursitis or tendon sheath inflammation can be easily diagnosed by locating tenderness/swelling/redness on palpation and eliciting the pain by tendon movement against resistance.

It is important to exclude a possible systemic disease. If there is clinical suspicion of underlying rheumatic disease, laboratory studies should be considered to evaluate the possibility of gout (hyperuricemia), rheumatoid arthritis (rheumatoid factor [RF]), and seronegative spondyloarthropathies (eg, human leukocyte antigen [HLA] B-27, erythrocyte sedimentation rate [ESR], C-reactive protein [CRP]).

Imaging

Imaging studies include weight-bearing X-rays of the ankle with anteroposterior, lateral and mortise views. X-rays of the foot may be obtained according to the symptoms and in specific conditions (e.g., rheumatic conditions, tarsal coalitions, pain extending to the foot), with weight bearing anteroposterior and lateral views, together with an oblique view. In case of hindfoot malalignment, a Cobey-Saltzman view may be obtained[6]. Traditional radiology is able to point out bone or cartilage conditions causing or mimicking bursitis (Figure 2), including: Haglund's deformity, exostosis, coalitions, tumors, osteochondral lesions, os trigonum, arthritis, etc.

In order to better evaluate the soft tissue and possible inflammation, ultrasound and/or MRI are also obtained. Tendinopathy (of the extensor, flexor, and Achilles tendons), increased synovial fluid in the bursae of tendon sheaths, chondral lesions, and stress fractures are clearly identified by MRI.

Conservative Treatment

The treatment of ankle bursitis begins with conservative treatment. It is mandatory for the patient to decrease the physical activity level.

Patients with bursitis should be instructed to ice the inflamed/tender area of the ankle and modify footwear. Orthotics like soft insoles with medial/lateral support (in case of malalignment) or silicone heel cups may be beneficial. Gradual stretching of the Achilles tendon and plantar fascia helps to decrease pressure on the retrocalcaneal bursa.

Other treatment options include the use of NSAIDs (local and/or systemic) or injections with corticosteroids. However, corticosteroid injections are not recommended in proximity of a tendon (due to the increased risk of tendon rupture [7]) or in the subcutaneous tissue (because of the risk of corticosteroid induced skin dystrophy). Therefore, in ankle bursitis corticosteroid injections are not recommended.

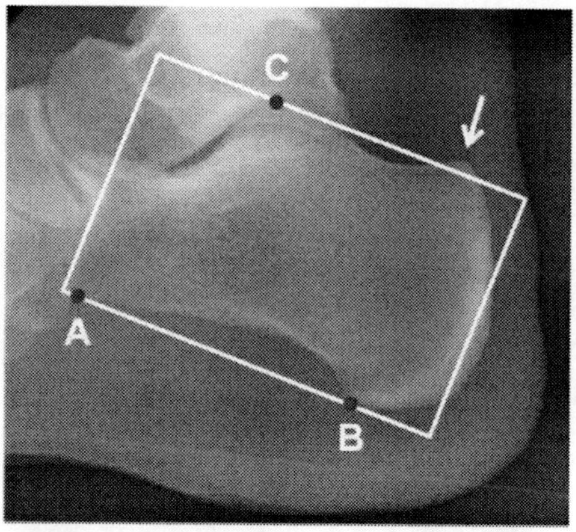

Figure 2. Lateral radiograph of the ankle demonstrating the parallel pitch line method for diagnosing Haglund's deformity. The first line is drawn from the anterior tubercle (A) to the medial tubercle (B). The second line parallels the first line and starts at the highest point of the posterior facet of the subtalar joint surface (C). Note that the tip of the posterior superior tubercle of the calcaneum (arrow) lies above the second line, pathognomonic of Haglund's deformity.

Most of the patients with superficial bursitis (subcutaneous Achilles, medial and lateral malleolus bursitis) do not require surgical treatments. On the other hand, about 15–50% of the patients suffering from chronic (more than 3 months) RB do not benefit from conservative management, mostly when Haglund's deformity is present, and consequently undergo surgical treatment [8].

Surgical Treatment

Resection of the retrocalcaneal bursa and Haglund's tuberosity is the main focus of operative treatment for RB [9]. This can be obtained either via open or endoscopy surgery. Open surgery requires large exposure with a consequent high risk of wound and soft tissue problems, especially in this anatomical area where the circulation is poor. Numerous studies and substantial progress have been made regarding arthroscopic/endoscopic ankle surgery [10]. Endoscopy has become an important mean in the treatment of numerous ankle, subtalar, and extraarticular pathologies, with the advantage of a quicker recovery and a shorter hospitalization compared with traditional open techniques. Despite the minimal invasiveness of the technique, arthroscopy is not free from complications. Posterior ankle/subtalar arthroscopy has a longer learning curve compared with anterior arthroscopy and should be performed by skilled arthroscopists. A thorough knowledge of the anatomy, correct indications, and a precise surgical technique are essential to achieve good outcomes.

The authors prefer an open surgical approach when debridement or repair of the Achilles tendon is necessary to treat marked degeneration or partial ruptures respectively.

On the other hand, an endoscopic approach is preferred when only bursectomy and Haglund's deformity resection is required. In case of initial Achilles tendon degeneration, an endoscopic approach with percutaneous longitudinal incisions of the tendon is preferred.

Open Surgery

General with a regional block or spinal anesthesia is performed. Pre-operative antibiotic prophylaxis is administered with Cefazolin 2 gr i.v. for adults and 30 mg/kg for children. The patient is positioned prone with the feet hanging off the operative table and adequate padding under head, chest, knees, elbows and shins. The tourniquet is positioned at the proximal thigh.

Traditionally, Haglund's deformity resection is performed through a posteromedial [11] or posterolateral [12] approach (Figure 3). A 4-5 cm skin incision is performed posteromedially or posterolaterally. The lateral approach is easier but care must be taken to avoid the sural nerve. The incision is vertical, 1 cm anterior to the Achilles tendon, starting from the posterior calcaneal tuberosity and extended proximally. The retrocalcaneal bursa is identified just anterior to the Achilles tendon and excised. The Haglund's deformity resection is performed with an oscillating saw or with chisels proximal to the Achilles tendon insertion. The excised bone is about 3 cm wide, 3 cm long, and 0.5-1 cm thick. The surfaces are then smoothened with a rasp or burr. In case of Achilles tendinopathy, the tendon can be partially detached from its insertion and debridement of the anterior degenerated tissue can be carried out. The tendon is then re-inserted back to the bone with suture anchors. Problems with lateral approach include poor deep visualization (e.g. it is difficult to reach the medial calcaneus from a posterolateral approach) and difficult Achilles tendon debridement.

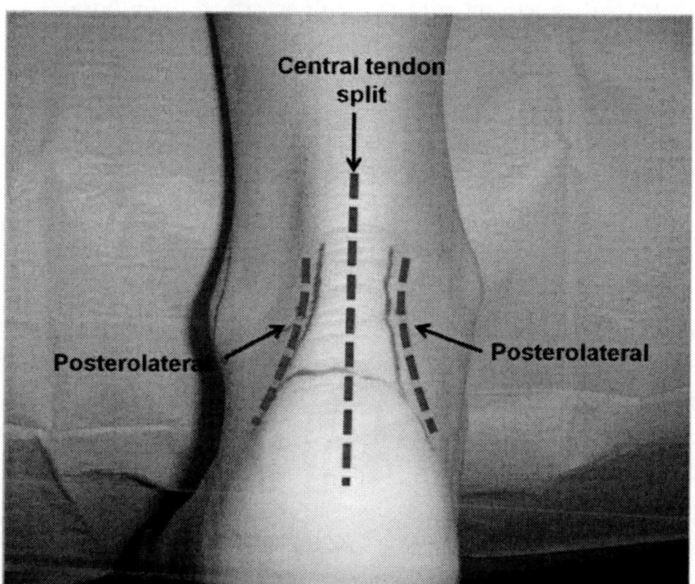

Figure 3. Possible open approaches for Haglund's deformity resection (see text).

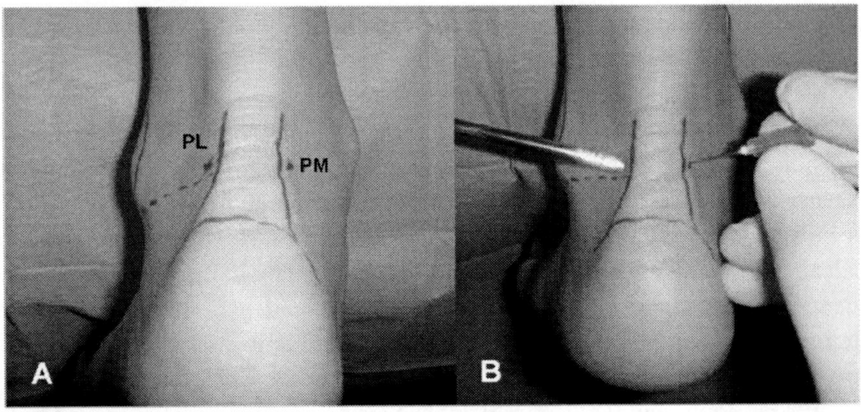

Figure 4. A) posterolateral (PL) and posteromedial (PM) portal placement. B) PL portal is placed first and then the PM portal is performed under direct visualization.

For these reasons a central Achilles tendon-splitting approach has been described. The patient is prepped and positioned as described before. The incision is centered over the Achilles tendon, from approximately 8 cm proximal to its insertion and extended distally to the glabrous skin (Figure 3). The central Achilles tendon-split is then performed longitudinal. The Achilles tendon insertion is partially detached (about 50%) in an *open book* fashion from central to lateral or medial, to better expose the Haglund's deformity and the degenerated anterior portion of the tendon. The bursa is then excised. All areas of fibrous degeneration and calcification of the tendon are removed with sharp dissection. The Haglund's deformity resection is performed with an oscillating saw and chisels and the bony prominences are smoothened as described before. The tendon is then reattached back to the bone with 2 or 4 suture anchors.

Independently of the approached used, the post-operative regimen includes a below-knee cast for 4 weeks followed by a boot for an additional 4 to 6 weeks. Range of motion exercises are begun at 4 weeks and toe-touch weight bearing at 6 weeks. At 8 weeks, full weight bearing is allowed. Physical therapy includes gastrocnemius and soleus muscle strengthening, as well as stretching exercises.

Comparable results have been described for the lateral approach and the tendon splitting. However, patients in the tendon-splitting group seem to return to normal function earlier than patients with the lateral approach [12].

Endoscopic Surgery

The patient is prepped and positioned as described before for the open procedures. Generally a prone positioned is preferred for posterior ankle and subtalar arthroscopies. However, when only excision of the RB and Haglund's deformity is planned, a supine position can be used with a bump under the hip (neutral position of the foot). The Achilles tendon and the medial and lateral malleoli are marked with a surgical pen (Figure 4). With the ankle in the neutral position, a line is drawn from the tip of the lateral malleolus to the Achilles tendon, parallel to the foot sole. The posterolateral (PL) portal is placed above this line, tangential to the Achilles tendon, and generally made first . A longitudinal PL skin incision is made and a blunt instrument is inserted toward the lateral aspect of the subtalar joint. A 2.7 or 4.5-mm 30°-angle arthroscope is then inserted into the lateral recess of the subtalar joint and the flexor hallucis longus (FHL) is visualized, as the arthroscope is moved medially. The FHL tendon is an important landmark and should always be kept in view medially, in order to avoid damage to the neurovascular bundle during the procedure. A needle is inserted into the joint at the level of the posteromedial (PM) portal, (tangential to the Achilles tendon, at the same level of the PL portal). The needle is visualized with the arthroscope to ensure it is lateral to the FHL (Figure 5). The PM portal longitudinal skin incision is then made. A mosquito clamp is bluntly introduced into the lateral aspect of the subtalar joint and directed toward the arthroscope. The clamp is used to spread the soft tissue in front of the arthroscope [13]. Synovium and fat pad are then removed with a shaver. The ankle and subtalar joints can be inspected and associated pathology can be treated if necessary. Excision of the RB is performed with the shaver until the Haglund's deformity is clearly visualized. This is then resected with a burr. Attention should be paid to perform adequate osteoplasty (fluoroscopy can help assessing the amount of bone removed). Percutaneous longitudinal puncture tenotomies can be used to treat initial degeneration of the Achilles tendon, when present.

Post-operatively, the patients are discharged the same day, with range of motion exercises and weight bearing as tolerated, in a post-operative boot for pain control. At 3 weeks from surgery, the boot can be discontinued and the patient advanced to full daily activities. At 6-8 weeks, the patient can be progressed to sports without restrictions.

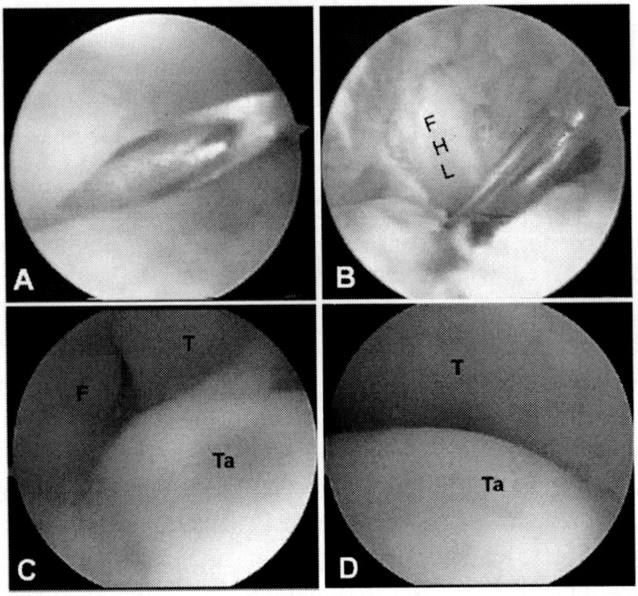

Figure 5. A) Needle insertion for PM portal placement. B) Visualization of the flexor hallucis longus (FHL). C) Lateral ankle view. D) Medial ankle view. T=tibia; Ta=Talus; F=Fibula.

Posterior arthroscopy has proven to be safe [14] and arthroscopic calcaneoplasty reported 95% of favorable outcomes [15]. In a recent systematic review, the different surgical treatment options for chronic RB have been evaluated. The authors concluded that, regardless of the technique used, resecting sufficient bone is essential for a good outcome. Even though the level of evidence of included studies is relatively low, it can be concluded that endoscopic surgery is superior to open intervention for RB. More evidence is necessary in order to be more conclusive regarding the best surgical treatment[3].

References

[1] Painter, CF. Inflammation of the post-calcaneal bursa associated with exostosis. *Trans Am Orthop Assoc*, 1898, 111(1), 169-180.

[2] Haglund, P. Beitrag zur Klinik der Achillessehne. *Zeitschr Orthop Chir*, 1928, 49, 49-58.

[3] Wiegerinck, JI; Kok, AC; van Dijk, CN. Surgical treatment of chronic retrocalcaneal bursitis. *Arthroscopy.*, 2012, 28(2), 283-93.

[4] Kachlik, D; Baca, V; Cepelik, M; Hajek, P; Mandys, V; Musil, V; Skala, P; Stingl, J. Clinical anatomy of the retrocalcaneal bursa. *Surg Radiol Anat.*, 2008, 30(4), 347-53.

[5] Reule, CA; Alt, WW; Lohrer, H; Hochwald, H. Spatial orientation of the subtalar joint axis is different in subjects with and without Achilles tendon disorders. *Br J Sports Med.*, 2011, 45(13), 1029-34.

[6] Saltzman, CL; el-Khoury, GY. The hindfoot alignment view. *Foot Ankle Int.*, 1995, 16(9), 572-6.

[7] Kleinman, M; Gross, AE. Achilles tendon rupture following steroid injection. Report of three cases. *J Bone Joint Surg Am.*, 1983, 65(9), 1345-47.

[8] Lohrer, H. Minimally invasive repair of an impingement induced partial tear of the anterior Achilles tendon in a top level athlete. *Z. Orthop. Unfall.*, 2010, 148, 80–82.

[9] Lohrer, H; Arentz, S; Nauck, T; Dorn Lange, NV; Konerding, MA. The Achilles tendon insertion is crescent-shaped: an in vitro anatomic investigation. *Clin. Orthop. Relat. Res.*, 2008, 466, 2230–37.

[10] Gasparetto, F; Collo, G; Pisanu, G; Villella, D; Drocco, L; Cerlon, R; Bonasia, DE. Posterior ankle and subtalar arthroscopy: indications, technique, and results. *Curr Rev Musculoskelet Med.*, 2012, 5(2), 164-70.

[11] Sammarco, GJ; Taylor, AL. Operative management of Haglund's deformity in the nonathlete: a retrospective study. *Foot Ankle Int.*, 1998, 19(11), 724-9.

[12] Anderson, JA; Suero, E; O'Loughlin, PF; Kennedy, JG. Surgery for retrocalcaneal bursitis: a tendon-splitting versus a lateral approach. *Clin Orthop Relat Res.*, 2008, 466(7), 1678-82.

[13] Bonasia, DE; Phisitkul, P; Saltzman, CL; Barg, A; Amendola, A. Arthroscopic resection of talocalcaneal coalitions. *Arthroscopy.*, 2011, 27(3), 430-5.

[14] Nickisch, F; Barg, A; Saltzman, CL; Beals, TC; Bonasia, DE; Phisitkul, P; Femino, JE; Amendola, A. Postoperative complications of posterior ankle and hindfoot arthroscopy. *J Bone Joint Surg Am.*, 2012, 94(5), 439-46.

[15] Van Dijk, CN; van Dijk, GE; Scholten, PE; Kort, NP. Endoscopic Calcaneoplasty. *Am J Sports Med.*, 2001, 29, 185–9.

Index

C

D

E

F

G

H

I

J

K

L

M

N

O

P

Q

R

S

T

U

V

W

X